Yoga Beyond 60

A Guide to Unlocking Vitality and Inner Peace for Seniors And Thriving in the Golden Years

Rishi Ashraf

Copyright © 2023 by Rishi Ashraf

All rights reserved.

No portion of this book may be reproduced in any form without written permission from the publisher or author, except as permitted by U.S. copyright law.

This publication is designed to provide accurate and authoritative information in regard to the subject matter covered. It is sold with the understanding that neither the author nor the publisher is engaged in rendering legal, investment, accounting or other professional services. While the publisher and author have used their best efforts in preparing this book, they make no representations or warranties with respect to the accuracy or completeness of the contents of this book and specifically disclaim any implied warranties of merchantability or fitness for a particular purpose. No warranty may be created or extended by sales representatives or written sales materials. The advice and strategies contained herein may not be suitable for your situation. You should consult with a professional when appropriate. Neither the publisher nor the author shall be liable for any loss of profit or any other commercial damages, including but not limited to special, incidental, consequential, personal, or other damages.

Book Cover by Eugo Grafix

1st edition 2023

Table Of Contents

Introduction	4
Benefits of Yoga for Seniors	6
Overview	15
Chapter 1: Getting Started with Yoga	19
Setting Realistic Goals	22
Choosing the Right Yoga Style	27
Modifications for Seniors	31
Essential Equipment and Props	37
Creating A Yoga Space	42
Chapter 2: Gentle Yoga Asanas (Poses) for Seniors	51
Warm-Up Exercises	54
Standing Poses	58
Seated Poses	64
Supine and Prone Poses	69
Balance Poses	74
Restorative Poses	79
Breathing Techniques and Mindfulness	84
Chapter 3: Yoga for Common Health Issues	92
Joint Stiffness and Flexibility	95
Arthritis and Joint Pain	99
Osteoporosis and Bone Health	102

Back Pain and Spine Health	106
Modifying the Practice for Specific Conditions	111
Seeking Guidance from Healthcare Professionals	115
Chapter 4: Yoga for Overall Well-being and Mindfulness	121
Stress Reduction and Relaxation	124
Mental Clarity and Focus	128
Emotional Well-being and Self-Awareness	132
Meditation and Mindfulness Techniques	136
Embracing Yoga Philosophy in Daily Life	140
Self-Care Practices for Seniors	145
Chapter 5: Maintaining a Yoga Practice	153
Establishing a Routine	155
Adapting the Practice as You Age	158
Continuing Education and Growth	162
Finding Supportive Communities	165
Conclusion	172

Introduction

"Yoga is the journey of the self, through the self, to the self."

- The Bhagavad Gita

Welcome to "Yoga Beyond 60"! In this book, we will explore the wonderful world of yoga and its incredible benefits for individuals in their golden years. Whether you are new to yoga or have practiced it before, this guide will provide you with valuable insights, practical advice, and a wealth of yoga practices specifically tailored for seniors.

Yoga is a time-honored discipline that encompasses physical postures, breath control, meditation, and philosophical principles. It is an ancient practice that offers numerous benefits for people of all ages, but it holds particular significance for seniors. As we age, maintaining flexibility, strength, and balance becomes increasingly important. Yoga provides a holistic approach to wellness that addresses these needs while nurturing the mind, body, and spirit.

The benefits of practicing yoga as a senior are truly remarkable. Regular yoga practice can improve your flexibility, enhance your balance, strengthen your muscles, and promote a sense of overall well-being. It can also help manage common health conditions that may arise with age, such as joint stiffness, arthritis, osteoporosis, and back pain. Moreover, yoga offers mental clarity, stress reduction, and emotional resilience, supporting a positive outlook and greater enjoyment of life.

It's important to note that before starting any exercise program, including yoga, it is advisable to consult with your healthcare professional. They can provide personalized advice based on your unique health profile and guide you through any necessary modifications or precautions.

In this book, we will guide you through the essentials of practicing yoga as a senior, from getting started to exploring gentle yoga asanas (poses) specifically designed for your needs. We will address common health concerns and provide you with techniques and modifications to adapt the practice to your individual circumstances. Moreover, we will delve into the broader aspects of yoga, exploring its impact on your overall well-being, mindfulness, and self-care.

Remember, yoga is not a competition; it is a journey of self-discovery, self-acceptance, and self-care. Each person's yoga practice is unique, and it should be approached with patience, kindness, and respect for your body's abilities and limitations. By embracing yoga, you are embarking on a path that offers physical vitality, mental clarity, and a deeper connection to yourself.

Get ready to embark on this transformative journey, where the beauty of yoga awaits you. Let us begin by exploring the fundamentals and discovering the joy of yoga for seniors above 60.

Benefits of Yoga for Seniors

As seniors, it's essential to prioritize our health and well-being. Engaging in regular physical activity is crucial for maintaining a vibrant and fulfilling lifestyle. Yoga, with its gentle yet powerful approach, offers a multitude of benefits for seniors. Let's explore the remarkable advantages that yoga can bring to your life.

Improved Flexibility

Yoga is renowned for enhancing flexibility, which tends to decrease as we age. The gentle stretching and lengthening of muscles in various yoga poses help improve joint mobility and increase range of motion. With consistent practice, you may find that everyday tasks become easier, and you experience greater freedom of movement.

Enhanced Balance and Stability

Balance is a vital aspect of senior well-being, as it helps prevent falls and related injuries. Yoga postures often involve balance and stability, such as standing poses or one-legged balances. These poses engage your core muscles, improve proprioception (the body's awareness of its position in space), and enhance overall balance and coordination.

Increased Strength

Maintaining muscle strength is crucial for seniors to support joint health and overall physical function. Yoga poses, including standing, seated, and weight-bearing poses, activate various muscle groups, promoting strength and stability. As you progress in your yoga practice, you may notice improved muscle tone and greater ease in performing daily activities.

Joint Health and Flexibility

Yoga can help alleviate joint stiffness and promote joint health. The gentle movements and stretches in yoga poses enhance blood circulation to the joints, nourishing them with nutrients and reducing inflammation. Additionally, yoga's low-impact nature makes it an ideal exercise for seniors, minimizing stress on the joints while improving their flexibility and range of motion.

Stress Reduction and Emotional Well-being

Yoga offers profound benefits for mental and emotional well-being. By incorporating breathwork, mindfulness, and meditation, yoga helps calm the mind, reduce stress, and promote relaxation. It activates the parasympathetic nervous system, triggering the relaxation response and aiding in stress management. Regular yoga practice can enhance your mood, foster a positive outlook, and improve overall emotional resilience.

Improved Respiratory Function

Yoga emphasizes conscious breathing techniques, known as pranayama, which can enhance respiratory function. Deep breathing exercises practiced in yoga help strengthen the respiratory muscles, improve lung capacity, and enhance oxygenation. This can have a positive impact on energy levels, cardiovascular health, and overall vitality.

Bone Health and Osteoporosis Prevention

As we age, bone density tends to decrease, making seniors more susceptible to conditions like osteoporosis. Weight-bearing yoga poses, such as standing poses and gentle backbends, help stimulate bone growth, enhance bone density, and reduce the risk of fractures. Yoga also promotes proper alignment and posture, which supports spinal health and reduces the likelihood of osteoporotic-related issues.

Mind-Body Connection

Yoga encourages the integration of mind, body, and breath. Through mindful movement, you cultivate a deeper awareness of your body, its sensations, and its capabilities. This mind-body connection can enhance your sense of embodiment, self-acceptance, and self-care. By nurturing this connection, you can develop a greater appreciation for your body and its wisdom.

Remember, these benefits are not limited to physical aspects but also extend to your overall well-being and quality of life. As you embark on your yoga journey, approach your practice with patience, compassion, and respect for your body's limitations. With consistent effort and an open mind, you can experience the transformative power of yoga in your senior years.

In the following chapters, we will delve deeper into the world of yoga, exploring the fundamentals, gentle yoga asanas (poses) specifically tailored for seniors, addressing common health concerns, and guiding you towards a more holistic and mindful approach to well-being. Get ready to discover the joy and rejuvenation that yoga can bring to your life!

Addressing Concerns and Misconceptions

Yoga is a practice that can benefit individuals of all ages and fitness levels, including seniors. However, it is common for concerns and misconceptions to arise when considering yoga as a form of exercise, especially for those in their golden years. In this chapter, we will address these concerns and dispel any misconceptions to help you approach yoga with confidence and clarity.

Concerns about Physical Limitations

One of the most common concerns seniors have is whether their physical limitations or health conditions will prevent them from practicing yoga. It is important to recognize that yoga is highly adaptable and can be modified to suit individual needs and abilities. Yoga instructors who specialize in teaching seniors are trained to offer modifications, props, and variations that accommodate a wide range of physical abilities. By working with a qualified instructor, you can safely and effectively practice yoga, even if you have limitations such as joint stiffness, chronic pain, or mobility issues.

Fear of Injury

Another concern that may arise is the fear of sustaining injuries while practicing yoga. It is essential to approach yoga with mindfulness, respect for your body, and an understanding of your own limitations. Start slowly and listen to your body's signals. Communicate any concerns or limitations to your yoga instructor, who can provide guidance and modifications to ensure a safe practice. Remember that yoga is non-competitive, and you should never push yourself beyond your comfort zone. With proper alignment, guidance, and a gradual progression, the risk of injury can be minimized.

Misconceptions About Flexibility

Some seniors may believe that they need to be flexible to practice yoga. However, flexibility is not a prerequisite for starting yoga—it is a result of consistent practice over time. Yoga poses are designed to gently stretch and strengthen the body, gradually increasing flexibility. Even if you have limited flexibility, you can still enjoy the benefits of yoga and improve your range of motion with regular practice. Flexibility is a journey, and with patience and dedication, you will witness improvements in your body's mobility and suppleness.

Overcoming Self-Doubt

Seniors sometimes doubt their ability to engage in physical activities due to age-related changes or societal expectations. It's important to recognize that yoga is a personal journey that is adaptable to your unique circumstances. Yoga is not about comparing yourself to others or meeting external standards. It is about embracing your body, honoring its wisdom, and working within your own limits. Let go of self-doubt and approach your yoga practice with self-compassion, knowing that you are taking positive steps towards enhancing your well-being.

Finding the Right Yoga Style

There are various yoga styles, each with its own emphasis and approach. As a senior, you may wonder which style is best suited for you. Gentle and accessible styles of yoga, such as Hatha yoga, restorative yoga, or chair yoga, are often recommended for seniors. These styles focus on gentle movements, breath awareness, and relaxation, making them suitable for all fitness levels. Explore different styles and attend trial classes to find the one that resonates with you and meets your specific needs.

Importance of Qualified Instructors

Working with a qualified yoga instructor who specializes in teaching seniors is highly recommended. A skilled instructor can provide personalized guidance, offer modifications, and ensure that you practice safely and effectively. Look for instructors who have experience working with older adults, understand the specific needs and challenges of seniors, and prioritize individualized attention. A supportive and knowledgeable instructor can address your concerns, answer your questions, and create a positive and inclusive yoga environment.

Remember, yoga is a practice that celebrates your body's abilities and encourages self-acceptance. By addressing concerns and dispelling misconceptions, you can approach yoga with confidence, knowing that it is a practice that can be tailored to your needs and bring you numerous physical, mental, and emotional benefits. In the next chapter, we will guide you through the essential aspects of getting started with yoga, helping you lay the foundation for a safe and fulfilling practice.

Overview

This is a comprehensive guidebook that aims to help seniors embrace the practice of yoga and experience its transformative benefits. It provides valuable insights, practical advice, and a wealth of yoga practices specifically tailored for seniors.

The book is divided into five chapters, each addressing crucial aspects of yoga for seniors. It begins by introducing the numerous benefits of yoga for individuals in their golden years and dispelling common concerns and misconceptions. The importance of consulting healthcare professionals before starting any exercise program is emphasized, ensuring that readers prioritize their safety and well-being.

The book then moves on to guide seniors through the process of getting started with yoga. It covers topics such as setting realistic goals, choosing the right yoga style, understanding modifications for seniors, and acquiring the necessary equipment and props. Additionally, it offers practical advice on creating a dedicated space for yoga practice at home, making it easier for seniors to incorporate yoga into their daily lives.

A significant portion of the book is dedicated to introducing gentle yoga poses specifically tailored for seniors. Step-by-step instructions, accompanied by clear illustrations or photographs, are provided to ensure proper alignment and safety. The chapter covers a wide range of poses, including warm-up exercises, standing poses, seated poses, supine and prone poses, balance poses, restorative poses, and breathing techniques. By practicing these poses, seniors can enhance their flexibility, strength, balance, and overall physical well-being.

The book also addresses common health issues that seniors may face and provides yoga-based approaches to manage and alleviate these conditions. It offers targeted yoga poses, sequences, and breathing exercises that promote joint health, alleviate joint stiffness, reduce arthritis pain, enhance bone density, and support spinal health. By incorporating these practices into their routine, seniors can experience relief and improve their overall quality of life.

Furthermore, the book explores the broader aspects of yoga beyond the physical realm. It delves into stress reduction, relaxation techniques, meditation, and mindfulness practices suitable for seniors. It encourages readers to embrace yoga philosophy in their daily lives, fostering a positive mindset, self-awareness, and self-care practices. By nurturing their mental and emotional well-being, seniors can experience a deeper sense of calm, clarity, and contentment.

Throughout the book, the importance of seeking guidance from qualified instructors and healthcare professionals is highlighted. It provides safety tips, modifications for various physical limitations, and suggestions for adapting the practice to ensure a safe and enjoyable yoga journey for seniors.

By the end of this book, readers will have a solid understanding of how to incorporate yoga into their lives. They will experience the physical benefits of improved flexibility, strength, and balance, as well as the mental and emotional benefits of stress reduction, relaxation, and mindfulness. This book serves as a trusted companion, offering practical guidance and inspiration for seniors looking to enhance their well-being and embrace the joy of yoga.

Chapter 1: Getting Started with Yoga

"Yoga is the fountain of youth. You're only as young as your spine is flexible."

- Bob Harper

Congratulations on taking the first step towards incorporating yoga into your life! In this chapter, we will guide you through the process of getting started with yoga as a senior. Whether you are completely new to yoga or have some prior experience, this chapter will provide you with the necessary tools, knowledge, and confidence to embark on your yoga journey.

Yoga is a practice that can be adapted to suit individuals of all ages and fitness levels, including seniors. It offers a holistic approach to physical fitness, mental well-being, and spiritual connection. By practicing yoga, you can experience improved flexibility, strength, balance, reduced stress levels, and a greater sense of overall well-being.

Getting started with yoga as a senior requires a thoughtful and intentional approach. It is important to set realistic goals, choose the right style of yoga that aligns with your needs and preferences, and understand how to modify the practice to accommodate any physical limitations or health concerns you may have. This chapter will provide you with the necessary guidance and information to help you navigate these considerations.

We will begin by discussing the importance of setting realistic goals when starting a yoga practice. By understanding your motivations and expectations, you can tailor your practice to meet your unique needs and aspirations. We will explore the various benefits of yoga for seniors, from improved physical fitness to enhanced mental clarity and emotional well-being.

Choosing the right style of yoga is an essential aspect of your journey. With a multitude of yoga styles available, we will help you navigate through the options and find a style that resonates with you. Gentle and accessible styles of yoga, such as Hatha yoga, restorative yoga, or chair yoga, are often recommended for seniors due to their emphasis on gentle movements, breath awareness, and relaxation.

Understanding how to modify yoga poses is crucial for seniors, as it allows you to adapt the practice to your unique physical abilities and limitations. We will explore modifications, variations, and the use of props that can make poses more accessible and safe. You will learn how to listen to your body, honor its limitations, and cultivate a practice that suits your individual needs.

Creating a dedicated space for yoga practice at home is another important consideration. We will provide practical advice on how to set up a comfortable and inviting space where you can engage in your yoga practice, free from distractions and interruptions. This will allow you to establish a consistent routine and fully immerse yourself in the transformative power of yoga.

Throughout this chapter, we encourage you to approach your yoga practice with patience, self-compassion, and an open mind. Yoga is a personal journey, and each individual's experience will be unique. Embrace the process of self-discovery, and remember that progress is not measured by comparison to others, but by the growth and transformation you experience within yourself.

By the end of this chapter, you will feel empowered and equipped to begin your yoga practice as a senior. You will have the knowledge to set realistic goals, choose the right style of yoga, modify poses to suit your needs, and create a supportive environment for your practice. Get ready to embark on an enriching and fulfilling journey of self-discovery through the practice of yoga!

Setting Realistic Goals

When embarking on your yoga journey as a senior, it is essential to set realistic goals that align with your abilities, needs, and aspirations. Setting goals can provide you with a sense of purpose, motivation, and direction in your yoga practice. By establishing clear and attainable objectives, you can track your progress, celebrate milestones, and experience a sense of accomplishment. Here, we delve into the importance of setting realistic goals and provide practical tips to help you on your path.

What Are Your Intentions?

Before setting goals, take a moment to reflect on why you are pursuing yoga as a senior. Is it to improve flexibility and mobility, reduce stress, enhance balance and stability, or cultivate a greater sense of overall well-being? Understanding your intentions will help you clarify your goals and focus your energy in the right direction.

Start with Small Steps

It's crucial to begin with small, achievable goals to build momentum and avoid overwhelming yourself. For example, your initial goal could be to attend two yoga classes per week or practice yoga at home for 10 minutes each day. Gradually increase the duration and frequency of your practice as you feel comfortable and more confident. Starting small allows you to establish a sustainable routine and enjoy the process of gradual progress.

Consider Your Physical Abilities

As a senior, it's important to consider your physical abilities and any limitations or health concerns you may have. Take into account factors such as joint stiffness, muscle weakness, or chronic conditions when setting your goals. Adjust your expectations and choose goals that are realistic and attainable within your current physical capabilities. Remember, yoga is a practice that can be modified to suit your unique needs and limitations.

Be Mindful of Your Energy Levels

Seniors may experience variations in energy levels throughout the day. Take note of when you feel most energetic and alert, and consider scheduling your yoga practice during those times. Setting goals that align with your natural energy patterns will enhance your ability to commit to and enjoy your practice. Remember to listen to your body and allow for rest and recovery as needed.

Embrace the Journey, Not Just the Destination

Yoga is a lifelong practice, and the process itself is as important as achieving specific goals. Embrace the journey, stay present, and focus on the experiences and lessons you encounter along the way. Rather than solely fixating on achieving particular poses or milestones, appreciate the growth, self-discovery, and transformation that occur within you through consistent practice.

Celebrate Milestones

Acknowledge and celebrate your progress along the way. Set smaller milestones that serve as markers of your achievements. Whether it's holding a pose for a few extra seconds, noticing improved flexibility, or experiencing increased calmness during meditation, take the time to appreciate these milestones. Celebrating your accomplishments boosts motivation, confidence, and a positive mindset.

Adapt and Adjust

As you progress in your yoga practice, you may find that your goals need adjustment. Your abilities, interests, and aspirations may evolve over time. Be open to revisiting and modifying your goals as needed. Regularly evaluate and reassess your objectives to ensure they continue to align with your current circumstances and desires.

Remember, the most important aspect of setting goals in yoga is to approach them with self-compassion and a non-judgmental attitude. Each person's yoga journey is unique, and there is no one-size-fits-all approach. Be patient with yourself, embrace the fluctuations, and enjoy the process of growth and self-discovery.

By setting realistic goals, you will create a roadmap for your yoga practice as a senior. You'll experience a sense of purpose, progress, and fulfillment as you work towards your objectives. Stay committed, be adaptable, and savor the transformative power of yoga in your life.

Choosing the Right Yoga Style

When exploring the world of yoga as a senior, it is essential to choose a yoga style that suits your needs, preferences, and physical capabilities. The wide range of yoga styles available may initially seem overwhelming, but with some guidance, you can find the style that resonates with you and supports your well-being. Here, we delve into the factors to consider when choosing the right yoga style and provide an overview of several styles well-suited for seniors.

Consider Your Physical Abilities and Limitations

As a senior, it is crucial to choose a yoga style that accommodates your physical abilities and limitations. Take into account factors such as joint stiffness, muscle strength, balance, and any specific health conditions you may have. Gentle and accessible styles of yoga that focus on slow, controlled movements and breath awareness are generally recommended for seniors. These styles prioritize alignment, adaptability, and modifications to suit individual needs.

Assess Your Goals and Intentions

Reflect on your intentions for practicing yoga. Are you primarily seeking physical fitness, stress reduction, improved flexibility, or a deeper spiritual connection? Different yoga styles emphasize different aspects of the practice, so aligning your goals with the inherent qualities of a specific style can enhance your experience. For example, if you prioritize relaxation and stress reduction, you may lean towards restorative yoga or Yin yoga. If you seek a more dynamic physical practice, you may explore Hatha yoga or Vinyasa yoga.

Explore Gentle and Accessible Yoga Styles

Several yoga styles are well-suited for seniors due to their gentle nature and emphasis on modifications. Here are a few styles to consider:

- **Hatha Yoga:** Hatha yoga is a gentle, foundational yoga style that focuses on breath control and holding poses. It is an excellent choice for seniors as it allows for individual modifications and encourages mindfulness.

- **Restorative Yoga:** Restorative yoga involves holding passive poses supported by props for extended periods. It promotes deep relaxation, stress reduction, and gentle stretching. This style is ideal for seniors looking to unwind, restore energy, and cultivate a sense of calm.
- **Yin Yoga:** Yin yoga targets the deep connective tissues and joints through passive, long-held poses. It enhances flexibility, increases circulation, and encourages a meditative state. Yin yoga can be particularly beneficial for seniors dealing with joint stiffness or limited mobility.
- **Chair Yoga:** Chair yoga modifies traditional yoga poses to be performed while seated or using a chair for support. It provides gentle stretching, improves flexibility, and enhances stability. Chair yoga is an excellent option for seniors with limited mobility or balance concerns.
- **Gentle Flow or Slow Flow Yoga:** Gentle flow or slow flow classes offer a relaxed and unhurried pace, combining gentle movement with breath awareness. These styles provide a balance of strength, flexibility, and relaxation, making them

suitable for seniors who enjoy a moderate level of activity.

Seek Guidance from Qualified Instructors

When choosing a yoga style, it is essential to seek guidance from qualified yoga instructors who have experience teaching seniors or modified yoga classes. Instructors who understand the unique needs and considerations of seniors can provide appropriate modifications, offer personalized guidance, and ensure your safety throughout the practice. Attend classes specifically designed for seniors or those with gentle or modified yoga options.

Try Different Styles and Listen to Your Body

The best way to find the right yoga style for you is through personal exploration and experimentation. Attend trial classes or workshops to experience different styles firsthand. Pay attention to how your body responds to different movements, the level of challenge, and how you feel mentally and emotionally during and after the practice. Your body's feedback will guide you towards the style that resonates with you the most.

Remember, there is no one-size-fits-all approach to choosing a yoga style. It is a personal journey that should align with your needs, preferences, and physical capabilities. Be open to exploring and adapting your practice as you evolve and grow. With the right yoga style, you can enjoy the multitude of benefits that yoga offers and embark on a transformative journey towards improved well-being as a senior.

Modifications for Seniors

As a senior practicing yoga, it is essential to embrace modifications that cater to your unique physical abilities, limitations, and overall well-being. Modifications allow you to adapt the poses and practices to suit your specific needs, ensuring a safe and enjoyable yoga experience. By understanding and utilizing modifications, you can fully engage in the practice, enhance your strength and flexibility, and promote overall health. Here, we explore the importance of modifications for seniors and provide practical tips to help you modify your yoga practice effectively.

Why Modifications Matter for Seniors

Modifications play a crucial role in the yoga practice for seniors, providing a multitude of benefits that contribute to their overall well-being. As we age, our bodies may experience certain limitations and physical conditions that require special attention and care. By incorporating modifications, seniors can ensure their safety and prevent the risk of injuries or strain during yoga sessions.

Safety is of paramount importance, and modifications serve as a safeguard, allowing seniors to practice yoga without compromising their well-being. Factors such as joint stiffness, reduced flexibility, or decreased balance can be addressed through appropriate modifications tailored to suit the body's capabilities. By adapting poses to their specific needs, seniors can engage in yoga confidently, knowing that they are taking necessary precautions to protect themselves.

Yoga is a practice that should be accessible and inclusive to individuals of all ages and physical conditions. Modifications make this possible, breaking down barriers and enabling seniors with varying abilities to actively participate in the practice. By adjusting poses to suit their specific requirements, seniors can fully experience the benefits of yoga and enjoy the sense of inclusivity within the yoga community.

One of the remarkable aspects of yoga is its ability to be tailored to individual needs. Each person's body is unique, and modifications allow seniors to personalize their practice according to their specific requirements. By making appropriate adjustments, they can experience the intended benefits of each pose while respecting their body's limitations. This individual tailoring ensures that seniors can engage in the practice at a level that is comfortable and beneficial for them.

In addition to customization, modifications also facilitate gradual progression in the yoga practice. It is crucial for seniors to honor their body's natural pace and avoid pushing beyond its limits. Modifying poses allows them to gradually build strength, flexibility, and balance over time. By embracing modifications and honoring their body's needs, seniors can foster a sustainable and progressive yoga practice that supports their overall well-being.

As seniors navigate their yoga journey, it is important to remember that modifications are not a sign of weakness or inadequacy. On the contrary, they are tools that empower individuals to honor their bodies and practice yoga in a way that is safe and beneficial for them. With the right modifications, seniors can engage in the practice confidently, experiencing the transformative power of yoga while respecting their unique physical circumstances.

By understanding the significance of modifications, seniors can approach their yoga practice with confidence, knowing that they have the tools to make the necessary adjustments. Modifications not only prioritize their safety but also promote accessibility, individual tailoring, and gradual progression. Seniors can embrace modifications as a means to embark on a fulfilling yoga journey that supports their physical, mental, and emotional well-being.

Tips for Effective Modifications

1. **Work with a Qualified Instructor:** Seek guidance from a qualified yoga instructor who has experience

teaching seniors or modified yoga classes. They can provide personalized advice, suggest appropriate modifications, and help you navigate your practice safely. An instructor can also provide hands-on adjustments and verbal cues to support your alignment and understanding of the modifications.

2. **Listen to Your Body:** Pay attention to how your body feels during the practice. If a pose causes discomfort or pain, it's essential to modify or skip that pose altogether. Be mindful of sensations, and honor what your body is telling you. Respect your limits and find variations that work for you.

3. **Use Props:** Props are valuable tools for modifying poses. Props such as blocks, straps, bolsters, blankets, or chairs can provide support, stability, and assistance in achieving proper alignment. For example, using a chair for balance or sitting on a block to elevate the hips can help make certain poses more accessible and comfortable.

4. **Focus on Alignment and Stability:** Modifications often emphasize proper alignment and stability to ensure a safe and effective practice. Pay attention to the alignment cues provided by your instructor and make adjustments accordingly. Engage your core

muscles to support your spine, maintain a steady breath, and cultivate a sense of stability throughout the poses.

5. **Reduce Range of Motion:** If you have limited flexibility or joint stiffness, it may be necessary to reduce the range of motion in certain poses. For example, in standing forward folds, you can bend your knees to ease the strain on the hamstrings. Adapting the poses to your body's capabilities allows you to experience the benefits without pushing beyond your limits.

6. **Modify Weight-Bearing Poses**: If you have concerns about balance or joint pressure, modifying weight-bearing poses can be beneficial. For instance, instead of performing a full plank pose, you can practice a modified version by placing your knees on the ground or leaning against a wall. This modification reduces the strain on the wrists, shoulders, and core muscles while still engaging in the pose.

7. **Embrace Restorative and Gentle Practices:** Restorative yoga and gentle yoga styles are particularly well-suited for seniors as they prioritize relaxation, gentle stretching, and stress reduction.

These practices often involve the use of props and longer holds in supported poses, allowing for deep rest and restoration.

Remember, modifications are not a sign of weakness but rather a way to honor your body's needs and capabilities. As you practice yoga, modifications may evolve and change. Be open to exploring different variations, and be patient with yourself as you adapt to new modifications. With time and consistent practice, you will discover modifications that best serve your body and support your well-being.

By embracing modifications, you can create a safe, inclusive, and enjoyable yoga practice as a senior. Modify poses as needed, listen to your body's wisdom, and experience the transformative power of yoga at your own pace.

Essential Equipment and Props

When practicing yoga as a senior, having the right equipment and props can greatly enhance your experience, support your body, and help you achieve proper alignment and stability. These tools provide assistance, modifications, and added comfort, making the practice more accessible and enjoyable. Here, we explore essential equipment and props that can be beneficial for seniors in their yoga practice.

Yoga Mat

A high-quality yoga mat is an essential piece of equipment for any yoga practice. Look for a mat that offers good cushioning and a non-slip surface to provide stability during poses. The mat should be thick enough to support your joints, especially if you have any knee or wrist sensitivities. Additionally, consider choosing a mat that is easy to clean and durable to withstand regular use.

Blocks

Yoga blocks are versatile props that provide support and stability, allowing you to modify poses according to your needs. They can be used to bring the floor closer to you, making poses more accessible and comfortable. For example, if you have limited flexibility, placing a block under your hand in a standing forward fold can relieve strain on the hamstrings. Blocks come in different sizes and materials, so choose ones that feel comfortable and provide adequate support.

Straps

Yoga straps are excellent tools for improving flexibility and reaching certain poses with ease. They assist in stretching and extending the reach of your arms when your flexibility is limited. Straps can be used to hold limbs in place during seated poses or provide assistance in deepening stretches. Opt for a strap made of durable material with an adjustable buckle or D-ring closure for easy adjustments.

Bolsters and Cushions

Bolsters and cushions are ideal for restorative and gentle yoga practices. They provide support and comfort, allowing you to relax and fully release into poses. Bolsters can be used to support the spine, hips, or legs, promoting relaxation and deepening the benefits of the poses. Cushions or meditation pillows offer added support and comfort during seated or reclined positions, allowing you to maintain a relaxed and upright posture.

Blankets

Blankets are versatile props that can be used in various ways during yoga practice. They can provide extra padding, support, or insulation. Folded blankets can be used to sit on and elevate the hips during seated poses, bringing the floor closer to you and reducing strain on the knees and hips. Blankets can also be used for additional cushioning or warmth during relaxation poses or to support the body in restorative poses.

Chairs

Chairs can be invaluable props for seniors with limited mobility, balance concerns, or specific physical conditions. Chair yoga is a modified form of yoga that incorporates the use of a chair for support and stability. It allows individuals to experience the benefits of yoga while sitting or using the chair as a prop for balance or modifications. Chairs provide a sense of security and can be used for seated poses, gentle stretches, or standing poses with support.

Eye Pillows or Masks

Eye pillows or masks are wonderful props to enhance relaxation and create a sense of calm during restorative or meditation practices. Placing a softly weighted eye pillow or a light-blocking mask over the eyes can help alleviate tension, promote relaxation, and aid in turning the focus inward. Choose ones made with soft and comfortable materials that allow you to fully immerse yourself in relaxation.

Additional Props

Depending on your specific needs and preferences, there are additional props that you may find beneficial in your yoga practice. These include foam rollers for self-massage and myofascial release, yoga wedges for added support and stability in poses, or even a yoga strap wall-mount for greater accessibility and support in stretching and strengthening exercises.

It's important to note that while these props can greatly enhance your yoga practice, they are not essential for every pose or practice. You can gradually build your collection of props as you explore different styles and variations of yoga. Additionally, attending classes or working with a knowledgeable yoga instructor can help you understand how to effectively utilize props to support your practice.

Investing in the right equipment and props can make a significant difference in your senior yoga practice. They provide support, modification options, and comfort, allowing you to adapt poses to your specific needs and capabilities. With the assistance of these props, you can enjoy a safe, accessible, and fulfilling yoga practice that nurtures your body, mind, and spirit.

Creating A Yoga Space

Having a dedicated space for your yoga practice can greatly enhance your experience, focus, and overall enjoyment of the practice. Whether you have a large room or a small corner, creating a yoga space that is inviting, peaceful, and tailored to your needs can make a significant difference in your senior yoga journey. Here, we explore essential considerations and practical tips for creating a yoga space that supports your practice and well-being.

Find a Suitable Location

Choose a location in your home that offers privacy, tranquility, and enough space for your yoga mat and movement. Ideally, select a room with natural light and good ventilation to create a fresh and uplifting atmosphere. If natural light is limited, consider adding soft lighting options or candles to create a calming ambiance.

Clear Clutter and Distractions

Clearing the space of clutter and distractions is crucial for cultivating a peaceful and focused environment. Remove any unnecessary objects or furniture that may hinder your movement or distract your attention. A clean and organized space promotes a clear mind and allows for uninterrupted practice.

Set the Mood

Consider incorporating elements that enhance the mood and ambiance of your yoga space. This can include soothing colors, calming artwork or photographs, inspirational quotes, or objects that hold personal significance. Choose items that resonate with you and create a positive and uplifting atmosphere.

Create a Sensory Experience

Engaging your senses can deepen your yoga practice and create a more immersive experience. Consider incorporating elements such as aromatherapy with essential oils, a small indoor water fountain for gentle sounds, or a soft music playlist to set the tone for your practice. Experiment with different scents, sounds, and textures to create a sensory experience that enhances your overall well-being.

Gather Essential Props and Equipment

Ensure that your yoga space is well-equipped with essential props and equipment. Keep your yoga mat, blocks, straps, bolsters, and blankets neatly organized and easily accessible. Having these props readily available encourages you to integrate them into your practice, supporting modifications, comfort, and stability.

Personalize with Plants and Natural Elements

Bringing elements of nature into your yoga space can add a sense of vitality and tranquility. Consider adding indoor plants, fresh flowers, or natural materials such as stones or seashells. These elements not only enhance the aesthetic appeal but also promote a connection with the natural world, fostering a deeper sense of grounding and harmony.

Consider Temperature and Ventilation

Maintaining a comfortable temperature and proper ventilation in your yoga space is essential for a pleasant practice. Ensure that the room is well-ventilated to allow for fresh air circulation. If necessary, use a fan or open windows to regulate the temperature during your practice. You may also want to have a blanket or shawl nearby for added warmth during relaxation poses or meditation.

Ensure Safety and Accessibility

Prioritize safety and accessibility in your yoga space, especially as a senior practitioner. Ensure that the flooring is even, non-slip, and free from tripping hazards. If necessary, use a yoga mat or non-slip rug to provide stability and traction during your practice. Consider adding handrails or wall supports for added stability during balance poses or if you have mobility concerns.

Create a Sacred Ritual

Establishing a ritual before starting your yoga practice can help you transition into a focused and present state of mind. This can include lighting a candle or incense, setting an intention, practicing a few minutes of mindfulness or deep breathing, or reciting a mantra or affirmation. Incorporate a ritual that resonates with you and helps you connect with the essence of your yoga practice.

Maintain Cleanliness and Organization

Regularly clean and maintain your yoga space to keep it inviting and energizing. Dust surfaces, wash your yoga mat, and tidy up after each practice. Keeping your space clean and organized not only contributes to a pleasant environment but also allows you to approach each practice with a fresh mindset.

Remember, your yoga space is a reflection of your inner sanctuary, a place where you can reconnect with yourself and find inner peace. By creating a yoga space that is tailored to your needs and preferences, you are establishing a supportive environment for your senior yoga practice. Embrace the opportunity to transform any corner of your home into a sacred space that nourishes your body, mind, and spirit, and allows you to fully immerse yourself in the transformative journey of yoga.

Conclusion

As you reach the end of this chapter on getting started with yoga, you have gained valuable insights into the foundational aspects of beginning a yoga practice as a senior. You have explored the importance of setting realistic goals, choosing the right yoga style, making modifications to suit your body's needs, and creating a dedicated yoga space. Now, armed with this knowledge, you are ready to take the first steps on your yoga journey.

Yoga is a personal and transformative practice that offers numerous benefits for seniors. By setting realistic goals, you can approach your practice with patience, kindness, and self-compassion. Remember that yoga is not about achieving perfection or comparing yourself to others. It is about embracing your unique journey and honoring your body's abilities and limitations.

Choosing the right yoga style is essential to ensure a practice that aligns with your needs and preferences. Consider gentle and restorative styles that prioritize relaxation, flexibility, and stress reduction. These styles provide a nurturing environment where you can cultivate strength, balance, and inner peace.

Modifications are a powerful tool that allow you to adapt poses and movements to suit your body. Embrace modifications as a way to prioritize safety, accessibility, and individual tailoring. Through modifications, you can make yoga poses more accessible, prevent injuries, and gradually build strength, flexibility, and balance.

Creating a dedicated yoga space is an invitation to cultivate a sanctuary where you can connect with yourself on a deeper level. Consider the elements that resonate with you—cleanliness, aesthetics, sensory experiences, and personal touches. This space becomes a reflection of your commitment to self-care, providing a supportive environment for your practice.

As you embark on your yoga journey, remember that it is a continuous process of self-discovery, growth, and self-care. Embrace the present moment, be mindful of your body's cues, and listen to its wisdom. Approach your practice with an open heart and an open mind, allowing the transformative power of yoga to unfold in your life.

Stay curious, explore different styles, attend classes, and connect with a supportive yoga community. Seek guidance from experienced instructors who can provide guidance, inspiration, and modifications tailored to your specific needs.

Yoga has the potential to enrich your life, enhance your physical well-being, promote mental clarity, and foster a deep sense of inner peace. Embrace the journey with patience, gratitude, and self-acceptance. With each breath, each movement, and each moment of stillness, you are nurturing your body, mind, and spirit.

Congratulations on taking the first step toward incorporating yoga into your life as a senior. Embrace the joy, the challenges, and the transformative power of this ancient practice. Trust in the process, and let the wisdom of yoga guide you as you embark on a path of self-discovery and holistic well-being.

Chapter 2: Gentle Yoga Asanas (Poses) for Seniors

In this chapter, we delve into the world of gentle yoga asanas (poses) specifically designed for seniors. As we age, our bodies undergo natural changes, and it becomes increasingly important to adapt our yoga practice to suit our evolving needs. Gentle yoga provides a nurturing and accessible approach, allowing seniors to experience the numerous benefits of yoga while honoring their bodies' unique requirements.

The practice of gentle yoga focuses on promoting flexibility, strength, balance, and relaxation. It emphasizes gentle movements, modifications, and mindfulness, creating a safe and supportive environment for seniors to explore their physical capabilities and enhance their overall well-being.

Throughout this chapter, we will guide you through a variety of gentle yoga asanas that are particularly beneficial for seniors. Each pose will be accompanied by detailed instructions, modifications, and considerations to ensure a safe and effective practice. Whether you are a beginner or have some experience with yoga, these gentle poses will help you cultivate strength, flexibility, and inner peace at your own pace.

One of the key principles of gentle yoga for seniors is the emphasis on modifications. We understand that each individual has unique physical limitations, such as joint stiffness, reduced mobility, or balance challenges. Modifications allow you to adapt poses to your body's capabilities, making the practice accessible and enjoyable.

The benefits of gentle yoga asanas for seniors are manifold. They promote joint mobility, improve flexibility, enhance muscular strength, and increase overall body awareness. Additionally, these poses can help alleviate common age-related issues such as arthritis, osteoporosis, and back pain. By engaging in a regular gentle yoga practice, you can experience improved posture, increased energy levels, reduced stress, and a greater sense of well-being.

It is important to approach these gentle yoga asanas with mindfulness and self-compassion. Listen to your body, honor its limitations, and practice within your comfort zone. Remember that yoga is a non-competitive practice, and comparison with others is unnecessary. Each pose is an opportunity to connect with your body, breath, and inner self.

As you embark on this exploration of gentle yoga asanas, we encourage you to create a calm and inviting space dedicated to your practice. Set aside any distractions, silence your phone, and allow yourself the time and space to fully immerse yourself in the practice. Utilize any props or modifications that support your comfort and stability, and remember that your yoga practice is unique to you.

Whether you are seeking to maintain or improve your physical well-being, reduce stress, or simply embrace a more mindful and peaceful lifestyle, gentle yoga asanas for seniors offer a holistic and transformative approach. With each pose, you have an opportunity to nourish your body, mind, and spirit, fostering a deeper connection with yourself and the present moment.

So, let us embark on this journey together, exploring the gentle yoga asanas that will support your health, vitality, and inner harmony as a senior practitioner. Open your heart and mind to the possibilities that lie ahead, and embrace the transformative power of gentle yoga for seniors.

Warm-Up Exercises

Warm-up exercises play a crucial role in any yoga practice, serving as the foundation for a safe, effective, and enjoyable experience. These exercises are designed to gradually awaken the body, increase blood flow, improve flexibility, and mentally prepare you for the physical and mental demands of yoga.

As a senior practitioner, incorporating warm-up exercises into your routine becomes even more essential. They help to lubricate the joints, reduce stiffness, enhance circulation, and minimize the risk of injury. Additionally, warm-up exercises provide an opportunity to connect with your breath, calm the mind, and transition from your daily activities into the focused practice of yoga.

In this section, we will explore a variety of warm-up exercises that are particularly beneficial for seniors. These exercises are gentle, accessible, and can be modified to suit your individual needs and abilities. Remember to approach each warm-up exercise with patience, attentiveness, and respect for your body's limitations.

Joint Mobilization

Begin your warm-up by gently mobilizing the major joints of your body. Start with the neck, slowly moving it in all directions—forward, backward, side to side, and in circles. Proceed to the shoulders, performing gentle shoulder rolls, backward and forward. Move on to the wrists, elbows, hips, knees, and ankles, gradually rotating and flexing each joint. This helps to improve joint mobility, increase synovial fluid production, and reduce joint stiffness.

Neck and Shoulder Rolls

Focus on releasing tension in the neck and shoulders with gentle rolls. Sit or stand with a relaxed posture, and slowly roll your shoulders backward in a circular motion. Coordinate this movement with your breath, inhaling as you roll your shoulders up and back, and exhaling as you roll them down and forward. Perform several rounds in both directions. Next, gently drop your right ear towards your right shoulder, allowing the left side of your neck to stretch. Hold for a few breaths and then repeat on the other side.

Spinal Warm-Up

Your spine is a vital part of your body, and warming it up is essential for a safe and effective yoga practice. Start by sitting on a chair or the floor with an upright posture. Place your hands on your knees and inhale deeply, lengthening your spine. As you exhale, slowly round your back, tucking your chin towards your chest. Inhale again and gently arch your back, lifting your chest and gazing up. Repeat this gentle cat-cow movement, coordinating it with your breath, for a few rounds. This warms up the spine, improves spinal flexibility, and awakens the core muscles.

Chest Opener

Sitting or standing with good posture, interlace your fingers behind your back, palms facing inward. Inhale deeply, expanding your chest, and gently lift your interlaced hands away from your body, feeling a stretch across the chest and shoulders. Hold for a few breaths, feeling the opening in your chest. Release and repeat a few times, remembering to maintain a relaxed and steady breath throughout.

Hip and Leg Circles

Sit comfortably on the edge of a chair or on the floor, extending one leg straight out in front of you. Slowly begin to rotate your foot in a circular motion, warming up the ankle joint. Then, move on to rotating your entire leg from the hip joint in large circles, first in one direction and then in the other. Switch legs and repeat. This exercise helps improve circulation, releases tension in the hips, and prepares your lower body for the standing and seated poses in yoga.

Deep Breathing and Mindfulness

Integrate deep breathing and mindfulness into your warm-up routine. Find a comfortable seated position, close your eyes, and take a few moments to connect with your breath. Inhale deeply through your nose, filling your lungs, and exhale fully, releasing any tension or stress. Focus your attention on the breath, observing its natural rhythm and sensation. This helps to center your mind, cultivate presence, and create a seamless transition into your yoga practice.

Remember, warm-up exercises are not meant to be strenuous or exhausting. Their purpose is to gently awaken and prepare your body for the upcoming yoga practice. Listen to your body, respect its limits, and modify the exercises as needed. By incorporating warm-up exercises into your routine, you set the stage for a safe, enjoyable, and fulfilling yoga experience as a senior practitioner.

Standing Poses

Standing poses are an integral part of a well-rounded yoga practice, providing a solid foundation for strength, stability, balance, and grounding. As a senior practitioner, incorporating standing poses into your routine offers numerous physical, mental, and emotional benefits. These poses help to improve posture, build lower body strength, enhance flexibility, increase circulation, and promote a sense of rootedness and confidence.

In this section, we will explore a variety of standing poses that are particularly beneficial for seniors. Each pose will be accompanied by detailed instructions, modifications, and considerations to ensure a safe and effective practice. Whether you are a beginner or have some experience with yoga, these standing poses will help you cultivate strength, stability, and inner harmony at your own pace.

Tadasana (Mountain Pose)

Begin by standing tall with your feet hip-distance apart. Distribute your weight evenly between both feet, grounding through the soles. Engage your leg muscles, lengthen your spine, and relax your shoulders down. Allow your arms to hang naturally by your sides with your palms facing forward. Breathe deeply and maintain a steady gaze forward. Tadasana helps improve posture, balance, and body awareness. It is an excellent starting point for all standing poses.

Modifications: If you have difficulty balancing, you can stand near a wall or use a chair for support. You may also widen your stance slightly to increase stability.

Warrior I (Virabhadrasana I)

From Tadasana, step your left foot back about 3-4 feet. Align your right heel with the arch of your left foot. Inhale and bend your right knee, keeping it directly above your ankle. Raise your arms overhead, reaching toward the sky, with your palms facing each other. Keep your torso facing forward and your back leg straight. Hold for a few breaths and then repeat on the other side. Warrior I strengthens the legs, opens the chest, and cultivates strength and focus.

Modifications: If you have knee issues, you can shorten your stance or bend your front knee to a comfortable degree. You can also keep your hands on your hips if raising them overhead is challenging.

Tree Pose (Vrikshasana)

Shift your weight onto your right foot and bring the sole of your left foot to rest on your right inner thigh or calf, avoiding the knee joint. Find your balance and bring your hands to a prayer position at your heart center. Lengthen your spine, relax your shoulders, and fix your gaze on a point ahead. Tree Pose improves balance, strengthens the legs, and promotes concentration and mental focus.

Modifications: If balancing on one leg is challenging, you can place the sole of your foot on the inner ankle or use a wall or chair for support. You may also lightly touch the toes of your lifted foot on the floor for added stability.

Extended Triangle Pose (Utthita Trikonasana)

Begin with your feet about 3-4 feet apart. Turn your right foot out 90 degrees and your left foot slightly inwards. Inhale and extend your arms to the sides, parallel to the floor. Exhale and reach your right hand forward, placing it on your shin, ankle, or the floor. Extend your left arm upward, creating a straight line from your left foot to your left hand. Gently turn your gaze upward or forward. This pose stretches the sides of the body, improves balance, and strengthens the legs.

Modifications: If reaching the floor or ankle is challenging, you can use a block or a chair for support. You can also shorten your stance or bend your front knee slightly to avoid strain on the hamstring or knee.

Chair Pose (Utkatasana)

Stand with your feet hip-distance apart. Inhale and raise your arms overhead, palms facing each other. Exhale and bend your knees, as if sitting back into an imaginary chair. Keep your weight in your heels, engage your core, and lengthen your spine. Hold for a few breaths, feeling the activation of your leg muscles. Chair Pose strengthens the thighs, tones the glutes, and improves balance and stability.

Modifications: If squatting deeply is challenging, you can sit on a chair with your feet hip-distance apart and practice the arm position. As your strength and flexibility improve, you can gradually reduce the chair height or perform the pose without the chair.

Mountain Pose Variation with Arms Swinging

Stand with your feet hip-distance apart and relax your arms by your sides. Inhale deeply, and as you exhale, swing both arms forward and upward, extending them overhead. Inhale again, and as you exhale, swing your arms back and down, bending slightly forward at the hips. Repeat this swinging motion, coordinating it with your breath. This variation promotes circulation, enhances shoulder mobility, and energizes the entire body.

Modifications: If you have any shoulder or balance issues, you can perform smaller swinging movements or hold onto a sturdy surface for support.

As with any yoga practice, it's important to approach standing poses with mindfulness and self-awareness. Listen to your body, honor its limitations, and practice within your comfort zone. Use props, such as a wall or chair, for support if needed. Remember that your yoga journey is unique, and each standing pose is an opportunity to connect with your body, breath, and inner strength.

Incorporating standing poses into your yoga practice as a senior practitioner offers a multitude of physical and mental benefits. They cultivate stability, strength, and balance while promoting a sense of grounding and confidence. By exploring these standing poses with patience, curiosity, and self-care, you can experience the transformative power of yoga in your daily life.

Seated Poses

Seated poses are an essential component of a comprehensive yoga practice, offering a wide range of benefits for seniors. These poses provide a stable foundation for cultivating flexibility, strengthening the core, improving posture, enhancing digestion, and fostering a sense of calm and inner awareness. Seated poses also allow for deeper exploration of the breath, mindfulness, and the integration of body, mind, and spirit.

In this section, we will delve into a variety of seated poses that are particularly beneficial for seniors. Each pose will be accompanied by detailed instructions, modifications, and considerations to ensure a safe and effective practice. Whether you are a beginner or have some experience with yoga, these seated poses will help you nurture your body, mind, and spirit with gentleness and compassion.

Easy Pose (Sukhasana)

Begin by sitting on the floor or a firm cushion, cross your legs, and place your hands on your knees or thighs. Find a comfortable position for your spine, aligning it upright without strain. If sitting on the floor is challenging, you can sit on a chair with your feet flat on the ground. Close your eyes or soften your gaze, and focus on your breath. Easy Pose promotes groundedness, flexibility in the hips, and encourages a calm and meditative state.

Modifications: If you experience discomfort in the knees or hips, you can place a folded blanket or cushion under the buttocks or sit on the edge of a folded blanket to elevate the hips slightly.

Seated Forward Bend (Paschimottanasana)

Sit on the floor with your legs extended straight in front of you. Inhale and lengthen your spine, then exhale as you fold forward from the hips, reaching towards your feet or ankles. Keep your spine long and avoid rounding your back. If reaching your feet is challenging, you can use a strap or hold onto your shins or thighs. This pose stretches the hamstrings, increases flexibility in the spine, and calms the mind.

Modifications: If you have tight hamstrings or lower back issues, you can bend your knees slightly or place a bolster or folded blanket on your thighs to support your upper body as you fold forward.

Bound Angle Pose (Baddha Konasana)

Sit on the floor with the soles of your feet together, allowing your knees to open out to the sides. Hold onto your ankles or feet with your hands. Sit up tall, lengthening your spine, and gently press your knees towards the floor. You can also add a forward fold, hinging from your hips, to deepen the stretch. Bound Angle Pose opens the hips, stretches the inner thighs, and stimulates the abdominal organs.

Modifications: If your knees are uncomfortable or do not reach the floor, you can place folded blankets or blocks under your thighs for support. You can also sit on the edge of a folded blanket or cushion to elevate the hips and reduce strain on the lower back.

Seated Twist (Ardha Matsyendrasana)

Sit with your legs extended in front of you. Bend your right knee and place the foot on the outside of your left thigh. Inhale and lengthen your spine, then exhale as you gently twist to the right, placing your left hand on your right knee and your right hand behind you for support. Look over your right shoulder. Hold the twist for a few breaths and then repeat on the other side. Seated Twist improves spinal mobility, massages the abdominal organs, and aids in digestion.

Modifications: If sitting with one leg crossed over the other is challenging, you can keep both legs extended and perform a seated twist by crossing one foot over the opposite thigh. You can also use a blanket or bolster for added support or sit on the edge of a folded blanket to elevate the hips slightly.

Half Lord of the Fishes Pose (Ardha Matsyendrasana)

Sit with your legs extended in front of you. Bend your right knee and place the foot on the outside of your left thigh. Inhale and lengthen your spine, then exhale as you twist to the right, bringing your left arm to the outside of your right knee and your right hand behind you for support. Look over your right shoulder. Hold the pose for a few breaths and then repeat on the other side. Half Lord of the Fishes Pose improves spinal mobility, stimulates the digestive system, and stretches the shoulders and hips.

Modifications: If sitting with one leg crossed over the other is challenging, you can keep both legs extended and perform a seated twist by crossing one foot over the opposite thigh. You can also use a blanket or bolster for added support or sit on the edge of a folded blanket to elevate the hips slightly.

Seated Meditation (Dhyana)

Find a comfortable seated position of your choice, either on the floor or on a chair. Close your eyes or soften your gaze, and bring your attention to your breath. Allow your body to relax, releasing any tension or tightness. Simply observe your breath and thoughts without judgment. You can also incorporate a mantra or positive affirmation during your meditation practice. Seated meditation cultivates mindfulness, clarity, and inner peace.

Modifications: If sitting on the floor is uncomfortable, you can sit on a chair with your feet flat on the ground. You can also use cushions, bolsters, or folded blankets to support your body and find a comfortable position.

Seated poses provide a nourishing and introspective aspect to your yoga practice. They encourage stability, flexibility, and inner awareness while fostering a sense of calm and tranquility. By incorporating these seated poses into your routine with mindfulness and self-care, you can tap into the transformative power of yoga and cultivate a deeper connection with yourself. Remember to listen to your body, respect your limits, and make any necessary modifications to ensure a safe and enjoyable practice.

Supine and Prone Poses

Supine and prone poses, also known as reclining and belly-down poses, play a vital role in a well-rounded yoga practice for seniors. These poses offer a unique opportunity to release tension, promote relaxation, rejuvenate the body, and develop core strength. They allow for deep rest and restoration while gently engaging and strengthening the muscles along the spine, abdomen, and back.

In this section, we will explore a variety of supine and prone poses that are particularly beneficial for seniors. Each pose will be accompanied by detailed instructions, modifications, and considerations to ensure a safe and effective practice. Whether you are a beginner or have some experience with yoga, these reclining and belly-down poses will help you find ease, support, and strength in your practice.

Supine Poses

Savasana (Corpse Pose)

Lie on your back with your legs extended and arms relaxed by your sides, palms facing up. Allow your body to fully relax into the ground, releasing any tension or effort. Close your eyes and bring your attention to your breath, letting it flow naturally and effortlessly. Savasana is a pose of complete surrender and relaxation, allowing the body and mind to rejuvenate and integrate the benefits of the practice.
Modifications: If lying flat on the ground is uncomfortable, you can place a bolster or folded blanket under your knees or use a rolled-up towel to support the natural curve of your lower back.

Supine Twist (Supta Matsyendrasana)

Lie on your back with your knees bent and feet flat on the floor. Extend your arms out to the sides in a T-shape. On an exhale, lower both knees to the right side, keeping your shoulders grounded. You can place a bolster or folded blanket between your knees for support. Gently turn your head to the left. Hold the twist for a few breaths and then repeat on the other side. Supine Twist releases tension in the spine, improves digestion, and promotes relaxation.

Modifications: If the twist feels too intense, you can place a folded blanket or bolster under your knees for support. You can also keep your top leg straight instead of bending it.

Bridge Pose (Setu Bandha Sarvangasana)

Lie on your back with your knees bent and feet hip-distance apart, heels close to your sitting bones. Press your feet into the ground, engage your glutes, and lift your hips off the mat. Interlace your fingers underneath your body, pressing your forearms into the ground. Keep your shoulders relaxed and draw your shoulder blades toward each other. Hold the pose for a few breaths and then slowly release down. Bridge Pose strengthens the glutes, hamstrings, and core muscles while opening the chest and hips.

Modifications: If lifting your hips off the ground is challenging, you can place a block or bolster under your sacrum for support. You can also perform a supported bridge by placing a block or folded blanket under your hips.

Prone Poses

Sphinx Pose (Salamba Bhujangasana)

Lie on your belly with your legs extended behind you and feet hip-distance apart. Place your forearms on the ground, parallel to each other, with your elbows under your shoulders. Press your forearms and pubic bone into the ground, engaging your core. Lift your chest and gaze forward, keeping your neck relaxed. Sphinx Pose strengthens the back muscles, improves posture, and stretches the abdomen and chest.

Modifications: If you have lower back issues or discomfort, you can place a folded blanket under your pelvis for added support. You can also lower your forearms to a comfortable height or practice a gentle variation by keeping your forearms on the ground and lifting only your head and chest.

Locust Pose (Salabhasana)

Lie on your belly with your legs extended behind you and feet hip-distance apart. Place your arms alongside your body, palms facing down. On an inhale, lift your chest, head, and legs off the ground. Keep your gaze forward and your neck in line with your spine. Engage your glutes and lift your legs higher. Hold the pose for a few breaths and then release down. Locust Pose strengthens the back muscles, improves posture, and stimulates the abdominal organs.

Modifications: If lifting both your chest and legs is challenging, you can start by lifting only your chest or legs individually. You can also use a folded blanket under your pelvis for added support.

Child's Pose (Balasana)

From a kneeling position, sit back on your heels and lower your forehead to the ground. Extend your arms in front of you or relax them alongside your body. Allow your entire body to relax and surrender to the ground. Child's Pose is a restful and grounding pose that releases tension in the back, shoulders, and neck while promoting a sense of peace and relaxation.

Modifications: If sitting on your heels is uncomfortable, you can place a folded blanket or bolster between your buttocks and your heels for support. You can also widen your knees or place a rolled-up towel under your forehead for added comfort.

Supine and prone poses provide a nurturing and rejuvenating aspect to your yoga practice. They offer a time for deep relaxation, release of tension, and development of core strength. By incorporating these reclining and belly-down poses into your routine with mindfulness and self-care, you can experience the profound benefits of both physical and mental rejuvenation. Remember to listen to your body, respect your limits, and make any necessary modifications to ensure a safe and enjoyable practice.

Balance Poses

Balance poses are an integral part of a well-rounded yoga practice for seniors. These poses not only improve physical balance but also cultivate mental focus, enhance body awareness, and foster a deep mind-body connection. By challenging equilibrium and stability, balance poses help seniors develop strength, coordination, and confidence.

Engaging in balance poses can be particularly beneficial for seniors as they enhance proprioception—the ability to sense the position and movement of the body. This is crucial for maintaining balance and preventing falls, which can be a significant concern for older individuals. Additionally, balance poses improve posture, increase joint stability, and build core strength, supporting overall physical well-being.

In this section, we will explore a variety of balance poses suitable for seniors. Each pose will be accompanied by detailed instructions, modifications, and considerations to ensure a safe and effective practice. Whether you are a beginner or have some experience with yoga, these balance poses will help you cultivate stability, focus, and a deeper mind-body connection.

Tree Pose (Vrikshasana)

Stand tall with your feet hip-distance apart. Shift your weight onto your left foot and bring the sole of your right foot to rest on the inner left thigh, above or below the knee. Find your balance and bring your hands together at your heart center or extend them overhead. Maintain a steady gaze on a fixed point in front of you. Tree Pose develops balance, strengthens the ankles and legs, and improves concentration.

Modifications: If placing your foot on your inner thigh is challenging, you can rest your foot on your calf or ankle instead. You can also use a wall or a chair for support until you feel more stable.

Warrior III (Virabhadrasana III)

Begin in a standing position with your feet hip-distance apart. Shift your weight onto your right foot, engage your core, and hinge forward at the hips. Simultaneously extend your left leg straight behind you, keeping it parallel to the ground. Extend your arms forward, palms facing each other or towards the ground. Maintain a strong and steady gaze at a fixed point. Warrior III strengthens the legs, improves balance, and enhances overall body awareness.

Modifications: If balancing on one leg is challenging, you can place your hands on a wall or a chair for support. You can also perform a modified version by bending your standing leg slightly or keeping your lifted leg closer to the ground.

Eagle Pose (Garudasana)

Stand tall with your feet hip-distance apart. Bend your knees slightly and lift your right leg, crossing it over your left thigh. If possible, hook your right foot behind your left calf. Bring your arms forward and cross your right arm over your left, bending your elbows to bring your palms together. Maintain a steady gaze and find your balance. Eagle Pose improves balance, strengthens the legs and ankles, and increases focus and concentration.

Modifications: If crossing your leg is challenging, you can rest the toes of your right foot on the ground or use a wall or a chair for support. You can also cross your arms at the elbows without binding them.

Standing Hand-to-Big-Toe Pose (Utthita Hasta Padangusthasana)

Stand tall with your feet hip-distance apart. Shift your weight onto your left foot and lift your right leg, bending the knee. Reach down and hold onto the big toe of your right foot with your right hand. Extend your right leg forward, keeping it straight if possible. Find your balance and keep a steady gaze. Standing Hand-to-Big-Toe Pose enhances balance, stretches the hamstrings, and strengthens the standing leg.

Modifications: If reaching your toe is challenging, you can use a yoga strap or a towel around the sole of your foot. You can also use a wall or a chair for support while extending your leg.

Modified Tree Pose (Vrikshasana)

Stand tall with your feet hip-distance apart. Shift your weight onto your left foot and place the sole of your right foot on the inner ankle, calf, or thigh—whichever feels most comfortable and stable. Bring your hands together at your heart center or extend them overhead. Find your balance and maintain a steady gaze. Modified Tree Pose provides stability and balance while reducing the demand on the hip joint.

Modifications: If placing your foot on your inner leg is challenging, you can rest your foot on your ankle or calf instead. You can also use a wall or a chair for support until you feel more stable.

Balance poses offer an opportunity to challenge and strengthen the body, cultivate focus and concentration, and deepen the mind-body connection. By incorporating these poses into your routine with mindfulness and self-care, you can improve your balance, stability, and overall well-being. Remember to listen to your body, respect your limits, and make any necessary modifications to ensure a safe and enjoyable practice.

Restorative Poses

Restorative poses are an essential component of a well-rounded yoga practice for seniors. These poses provide deep relaxation, healing, and renewal for the body, mind, and spirit. They are designed to release tension, reduce stress, and promote a state of calm and tranquility. Restorative poses are especially beneficial for seniors as they support the body's natural healing processes, aid in pain management, and enhance overall well-being.

In restorative yoga, the emphasis is on slowing down, gentle stretching, and using supportive props to create a nurturing and comfortable environment. The poses are typically held for an extended period, allowing the body to fully relax and surrender. Restorative poses help activate the parasympathetic nervous system, which promotes deep rest and relaxation, lowers blood pressure, and reduces stress hormone levels.

In this section, we will explore a variety of restorative poses suitable for seniors. Each pose will be accompanied by detailed instructions, modifications, and considerations to ensure a safe and rejuvenating practice. Whether you are a beginner or have some experience with yoga, incorporating restorative poses into your routine will allow you to experience deep relaxation, restoration, and healing.

Supported Child's Pose (Balasana)

Start by kneeling on the ground with your knees hip-distance apart. Place a bolster or a stack of folded blankets in front of you. Extend your arms forward and lower your torso onto the bolster or blankets, resting your forehead on the support. Allow your entire body to relax, releasing any tension or effort. Supported Child's Pose gently stretches the hips, back, and shoulders while inducing a sense of comfort and calm.

Modifications: If kneeling is uncomfortable, you can place a folded blanket or bolster between your buttocks and your heels for added support. You can also widen your knees or use additional blankets or cushions to adjust the height and support of the bolster.

Supported Reclining Bound Angle Pose (Supta Baddha Konasana)

Sit on the ground with your legs extended in front of you. Place a bolster or a stack of folded blankets behind you. Bend your knees and bring the soles of your feet together, allowing your knees to fall open to the sides. Lie back on the bolster or blankets, ensuring that your spine is fully supported. You can place additional blankets or cushions under your knees and thighs for added comfort. Close your eyes and allow your body to relax deeply. Supported Reclining Bound Angle Pose opens the hips, chest, and shoulders while promoting relaxation and surrender.

Modifications: If your hips are tight or if lying flat on the ground is uncomfortable, you can place additional blankets or bolsters under your thighs to elevate the legs. You can also place rolled-up blankets or towels under your outer thighs for support.

Legs-Up-The-Wall Pose (Viparita Karani)

Sit sideways next to a wall with your hip against it. Lie down on your back and extend your legs up the wall. Adjust your distance from the wall so that your legs are comfortably supported. You can place a folded blanket or a bolster under your hips for added support. Rest your arms by your sides or place your hands on your belly. Close your eyes and relax deeply. Legs-Up-The-Wall Pose promotes circulation, relieves swollen ankles, and rejuvenates the legs while inducing a sense of calm and relaxation.

Modifications: If you have difficulty reaching the wall or if it feels uncomfortable, you can use a chair instead. Place your legs on the seat of the chair, ensuring that your hips and lower back are supported. You can also place a folded blanket or bolster under your hips for added comfort.

Supported Supine Twist

Lie on your back with your knees bent and feet hip-distance apart. Shift your hips slightly to the right and extend your arms out to the sides in a T-shape. On an exhale, lower both knees to the left side, allowing them to rest on a bolster or stacked blankets. Gently turn your head to the right. Close your eyes and relax into the twist, feeling the gentle stretch in your spine and torso. Supported Supine Twist releases tension in the back, massages the internal organs, and promotes relaxation and detoxification.

Modifications: If the height of the bolster or blankets is too intense, you can reduce the height or use fewer layers of support. You can also place a folded blanket between your knees for added comfort and support.

Restorative poses offer a sanctuary of deep relaxation, healing, and renewal. By incorporating these poses into your practice, you can experience profound rest, stress reduction, and rejuvenation. Remember to create a comfortable and supportive environment with the use of props, listen to your body, and honor your limits. Allow yourself to fully surrender and embrace the healing benefits of restorative yoga.

Breathing Techniques and Mindfulness

Breathing techniques, also known as pranayama, are an integral part of yoga practice for seniors. They offer a powerful tool for managing stress, promoting relaxation, and cultivating a deep sense of calmness, clarity, and connection. Incorporating specific breathing techniques into your yoga practice can enhance the benefits of physical postures, deepen your mind-body connection, and bring a greater sense of well-being.

As we age, our breathing patterns may become shallower, and we may experience decreased lung capacity. Engaging in intentional breathing exercises can help expand the lungs, increase oxygen intake, and improve overall respiratory function. Breathing techniques also activate the parasympathetic nervous system, which helps counteract the effects of stress, reduce anxiety, and promote a state of relaxation and mental clarity.

Mindfulness, often combined with conscious breathing, is another key component of yoga practice for seniors. It involves paying attention to the present moment with non-judgmental awareness, fully immersing ourselves in the experience. By cultivating mindfulness, we can enhance our ability to stay present, reduce distractions, and deepen our connection to ourselves and the world around us.

In this section, we will explore various breathing techniques and mindfulness practices suitable for seniors. Each technique will be accompanied by detailed instructions, benefits, and considerations to ensure a safe and effective practice. By incorporating these techniques into your yoga routine, you can cultivate a greater sense of calmness, clarity, and connection.

Deep Belly Breathing

Deep belly breathing, also known as diaphragmatic breathing, is a foundational breathing technique that promotes relaxation and reduces stress. Start by finding a comfortable seated or lying position. Place one hand on your abdomen and the other on your chest. Take a deep breath in through your nose, allowing your abdomen to rise as you fill your lungs with air. Exhale slowly through your nose, feeling your abdomen gently contract. Continue this slow, deep breathing, focusing on the movement of your belly. Deep belly breathing helps activate the relaxation response, reduces anxiety, and enhances overall well-being.

Alternate Nostril Breathing (Nadi Shodhana)

Sit comfortably with your spine erect. Bring your right hand up and fold your index and middle fingers toward your palm, leaving your thumb, ring finger, and pinky finger extended. Use your thumb to gently close your right nostril and inhale through your left nostril. Close your left nostril with your ring finger, release your thumb, and exhale through your right nostril. Inhale through your right nostril, close it with your thumb, release your ring finger, and exhale through your left nostril. Continue this alternating breath pattern, moving at your own pace. Alternate nostril breathing balances the flow of energy in the body, calms the mind, and enhances mental focus and clarity.

Box Breathing (Square Breathing)

Find a comfortable seated position and relax your body. Inhale slowly and deeply through your nose for a count of four. Hold your breath for a count of four. Exhale slowly and completely through your nose for a count of four. Hold your breath again for a count of four. Repeat this box breathing pattern several times, maintaining a steady rhythm. Box breathing helps regulate the breath, calm the nervous system, and promote a sense of balance and tranquility.

Box Breathing (Square Breathing)

Find a comfortable seated position and relax your body. Inhale slowly and deeply through your nose for a count of four. Hold your breath for a count of four. Exhale slowly and completely through your nose for a count of four. Hold your breath again for a count of four. Repeat this box breathing pattern several times, maintaining a steady rhythm. Box breathing helps regulate the breath, calm the nervous system, and promote a sense of balance and tranquility.

Mindful Body Scan

Lie down in a comfortable position, close your eyes, and bring your awareness to your body. Begin by focusing on your toes and gradually move your attention up through your feet, ankles, calves, and so on, all the way up to the top of your head. Notice any sensations, tensions, or areas of relaxation in each part of your body. Stay present and non-judgmental, simply observing the sensations without trying to change them. The mindful body scan promotes deep relaxation, body awareness, and a sense of connection between the body and mind.

Loving-Kindness Meditation

Find a comfortable seated position and close your eyes. Take a few deep breaths to center yourself. Begin by directing thoughts of loving-kindness toward yourself, silently repeating phrases such as "May I be happy, may I be healthy, may I be safe, may I live with ease." After a few minutes, extend these thoughts of well-being to others, starting with a loved one, then to acquaintances, and eventually to all beings. Allow feelings of love, compassion, and kindness to arise as you cultivate a sense of connection and well-wishing for yourself and others. Loving-kindness meditation fosters positive emotions, empathy, and a sense of interconnectedness with all beings.

By incorporating these breathing techniques and mindfulness practices into your yoga routine, you can cultivate a deep sense of calmness, clarity, and connection. Remember to approach these practices with patience, curiosity, and self-compassion. As you explore the power of your breath and embrace mindfulness, you will discover a profound source of well-being and inner peace.

Conclusion

The practice of gentle yoga asanas for seniors offers a multitude of benefits for the body, mind, and spirit. Throughout this chapter, we have explored various categories of poses, including warm-up exercises, standing poses, seated poses, supine and prone poses, balance poses, and restorative poses. Each category provides unique advantages and contributes to a well-rounded yoga practice tailored specifically for seniors.

By incorporating these gentle yoga poses into your routine, you can improve flexibility, strength, balance, and overall physical well-being. The poses are designed to be accessible and adaptable, allowing you to modify and customize them based on your individual needs and capabilities. It's important to approach the practice with patience, listen to your body, and honor its limits. By doing so, you can experience the transformative power of yoga while minimizing the risk of injury or strain.

Furthermore, the practice of gentle yoga asanas extends beyond the physical benefits. It offers an opportunity to cultivate mindfulness, connect with the breath, and deepen the mind-body connection. Breathing techniques and mindfulness practices, such as deep belly breathing, alternate nostril breathing, box breathing, mindful body scans, and loving-kindness meditation, enhance the overall yoga experience, promoting relaxation, mental clarity, and a sense of inner peace.

Remember that yoga is a personal journey, and it's important to approach it with self-compassion and non-judgment. Embrace your unique abilities and limitations, and celebrate the progress you make on your mat, no matter how small. With regular practice, patience, and a gentle approach, you can experience the profound benefits of yoga at any age.

As we conclude this chapter on gentle yoga asanas for seniors, I encourage you to continue exploring and incorporating these poses into your practice. Embrace the joy of movement, the power of breath, and the serenity of mindfulness. Allow yoga to be a source of strength, vitality, and well-being in your life, and may it support you on your journey to a healthier, more balanced, and fulfilling life.

Chapter 3: Yoga for Common Health Issues

"Yoga is not about touching your toes, it's about what you learn on the way down."

- Judith Hanson Lasater

Yoga is a centuries-old practice that offers a multitude of benefits for the body, mind, and spirit. Its gentle and holistic approach makes it an ideal practice for addressing common health issues that seniors may encounter. From joint stiffness and arthritis to stress and anxiety, yoga provides a comprehensive framework for managing and improving various physical and mental conditions.

In this chapter, we will explore the transformative potential of yoga for common health issues that seniors often face. We will delve into specific health concerns, discuss how yoga can be beneficial, and provide a range of yoga poses, breathing techniques, and mindfulness practices that can support and enhance well-being.

Yoga offers a unique combination of physical movement, breathwork, and mindfulness, creating a holistic approach to health and healing. The gentle stretching, strengthening, and balancing of the body through yoga poses help improve flexibility, joint mobility, muscle strength, and overall physical well-being. Moreover, the mindful and meditative aspects of yoga help reduce stress, promote relaxation, enhance mental clarity, and cultivate emotional resilience.

Throughout this chapter, we will focus on addressing common health issues such as arthritis, osteoporosis, hypertension, back pain, stress, and anxiety. We will provide specific yoga poses and practices that are known to be beneficial for each condition. These poses will be accompanied by detailed instructions, modifications, and considerations to ensure a safe and effective practice tailored to your individual needs.

It is important to note that yoga is not a substitute for medical treatment or professional advice. If you have any underlying health conditions or concerns, it is essential to consult with your healthcare provider before starting a yoga practice. They can provide valuable insights, offer specific modifications based on your condition, and ensure that yoga complements your overall healthcare plan.

Yoga is a personal journey, and it is essential to approach it with self-compassion, patience, and an open mind. Each person's experience with yoga will be unique, and it is important to listen to your body, honor its limitations, and modify the poses and practices as needed. Yoga is not about achieving the perfect pose; it is about cultivating awareness, embracing self-care, and nurturing your body and mind.

As we embark on this exploration of yoga for common health issues, I invite you to open yourself to the healing power of yoga. Embrace the opportunity to discover new ways to support your well-being, enhance your quality of life, and find a deeper connection to yourself. May this chapter serve as a guide and inspiration as you incorporate yoga into your daily life, fostering a healthier and more balanced existence.

Joint Stiffness and Flexibility

Joint stiffness is a common issue that many seniors experience as they age. It can affect various joints in the body, such as the knees, hips, shoulders, and wrists, leading to discomfort, limited range of motion, and reduced flexibility. Fortunately, yoga offers a gentle and effective approach to address joint stiffness, promote flexibility, and restore fluidity of movement.

Yoga poses are designed to gently stretch and strengthen the muscles and tissues surrounding the joints. Through regular practice, yoga can help increase joint mobility, improve flexibility, and alleviate stiffness. The combination of movement, breathwork, and mindfulness in yoga provides a comprehensive approach to support the health and function of your joints.

Here are some key ways in which yoga can help with joint stiffness and promote flexibility:

1. **Gentle Stretching:** Yoga poses gently stretch the muscles and connective tissues around the joints, promoting lengthening and relaxation. This can help alleviate stiffness and improve joint mobility. Poses such as Forward Fold (Uttanasana), Standing Side Stretch (Parsva Uttanasana), and Seated Forward Bend (Paschimottanasana) are particularly beneficial for stretching the hamstrings, lower back, and hips.
2. **Range of Motion Exercises:** Yoga incorporates movements that take joints through their full range of motion. This helps lubricate the joints, increase synovial fluid production, and reduce stiffness. Poses such as Shoulder Rolls, Wrist Circles, and Ankle Rotations can help improve joint mobility and relieve stiffness in specific areas.
3. **Strengthening Supporting Muscles:** Strong muscles surrounding the joints provide stability and support, reducing strain on the joints themselves. Yoga poses focus on building strength in the muscles that support the joints, such as the

quadriceps, glutes, core muscles, and upper back muscles. Poses like Warrior II (Virabhadrasana II), Bridge Pose (Setu Bandhasana), and Plank Pose (Phalakasana) are effective for strengthening these areas.

4. **Mindful Movement:** Mindfulness plays a crucial role in yoga practice. By cultivating awareness of your body and its sensations, you can tune in to areas of tension, stiffness, or discomfort. Mindful movement allows you to approach your practice with sensitivity, honoring your body's limits and adapting poses to suit your needs. It helps you find a balance between effort and ease, avoiding overexertion and potential strain on the joints.

5. **Modifications and Props:** Yoga offers a wide range of modifications and props that can be used to adapt poses and make them more accessible for those with joint stiffness. Using props like blocks, blankets, or straps can provide support, stability, and a safe range of motion. Modifying poses by adjusting the depth or intensity can also help accommodate individual needs and limitations.

It is important to approach yoga for joint stiffness with patience, consistency, and an understanding that progress may be gradual. Remember to listen to your body and respect its limitations. Avoid pushing yourself into painful or uncomfortable positions. Instead, focus on finding a balance between challenge and comfort, gradually working towards increased flexibility and freedom of movement.

Incorporating yoga into your daily routine can bring significant improvements in joint mobility, flexibility, and overall well-being. By embracing the fluidity and freedom of movement that yoga offers, you can reclaim a sense of ease, reduce joint stiffness, and enhance your quality of life. Consult with a qualified yoga instructor or therapist to guide you in selecting appropriate poses and sequences tailored to your specific needs. With time and dedication, you can experience the transformative power of yoga in addressing joint stiffness and promoting flexibility.

Arthritis and Joint Pain

Arthritis is a common condition that affects the joints, causing pain, inflammation, stiffness, and reduced mobility. It can significantly impact the daily lives of seniors, limiting their activities and diminishing their quality of life. While there is no cure for arthritis, yoga offers a holistic approach to managing symptoms, improving joint function, and reducing pain.

Yoga is an ideal practice for individuals with arthritis due to its gentle, low-impact nature. It focuses on gentle movements, joint mobilization, strengthening, and stretching, all of which can provide relief and support for arthritis-related joint pain. Moreover, the mindfulness aspect of yoga helps cultivate a positive mindset, reduce stress, and improve overall well-being.

Below are some key ways in which yoga can help with arthritis and joint pain:

1. **Gentle Movement:** Yoga incorporates gentle movements that help increase joint mobility and decrease stiffness. The fluid and controlled motions

in yoga poses help lubricate the joints, promoting synovial fluid production and reducing friction. Slow and deliberate movements allow for gentle stretching and strengthening of the muscles surrounding the affected joints.
2. **Range of Motion Exercises:** Yoga poses emphasize taking joints through their full range of motion. This helps improve joint flexibility, reduce stiffness, and increase blood flow to the affected areas. Poses such as Cat-Cow Stretch, Knee-to-Chest Pose, and Gentle Spinal Twists can be particularly beneficial for improving joint mobility and relieving stiffness.
3. **Strengthening and Stability:** Yoga poses focus on strengthening the muscles that support the joints, providing stability and reducing strain on the affected areas. Strengthening exercises help maintain joint integrity, improve balance, and reduce the risk of falls. Poses such as Warrior I and II, Tree Pose, and Chair Pose help strengthen the legs, hips, and core muscles, providing support for the affected joints.
4. **Pain Management**: Yoga can help manage pain associated with arthritis through various techniques.

The practice of mindfulness and breathwork during yoga helps shift the focus away from pain and cultivates a sense of relaxation. Additionally, certain breathing exercises, such as Deep Belly Breathing and Progressive Muscle Relaxation, can help reduce pain perception and induce a state of calm.

5. **Stress Reduction:** Stress can exacerbate arthritis symptoms and contribute to pain and inflammation. Yoga's emphasis on mindfulness, deep breathing, and relaxation techniques helps reduce stress levels, promoting a sense of calmness and well-being. Stress reduction also positively impacts the immune system, which can play a role in managing arthritis symptoms.

It is important to approach yoga for arthritis with guidance and supervision, especially if you are new to the practice or have severe joint pain. Consulting with a qualified yoga instructor or therapist who has experience working with individuals with arthritis can provide valuable guidance on appropriate poses, modifications, and adaptations tailored to your specific needs.

Remember to listen to your body and practice self-care. If a pose causes pain or discomfort, modify it or skip it altogether. Focus on finding a balance between challenge and comfort, working within your personal limitations. Regular and consistent practice is key to experiencing the benefits of yoga for arthritis.

By incorporating yoga into your daily routine, you can find relief from arthritis-related joint pain, improve joint mobility, strengthen supporting muscles, and enhance your overall well-being. Embrace the healing potential of yoga, and allow it to become a source of support and empowerment on your journey to managing arthritis and reclaiming a fulfilling and active lifestyle.

Osteoporosis and Bone Health

Osteoporosis is a condition characterized by low bone density and deterioration of bone tissue, leading to an increased risk of fractures. It primarily affects older adults, especially postmenopausal women, and can significantly impact mobility and quality of life. While medical interventions are crucial in managing osteoporosis, incorporating yoga into your routine can play a complementary role in improving bone health, enhancing balance, and reducing the risk of falls and fractures.

Yoga provides a gentle yet effective approach to strengthen bones, improve posture, and enhance overall bone health. The weight-bearing nature of many yoga poses, combined with mindful movements and controlled breathing, can help stimulate bone remodeling, increase bone density, and improve bone strength. Additionally, yoga promotes balance, flexibility, and coordination, which are essential for preventing falls and fractures.

Here are some ways in which yoga can help with osteoporosis and promote bone health:

1. **Weight-Bearing Poses:** Weight-bearing exercises are beneficial for improving bone density. Yoga poses such as Warrior II, Tree Pose, and Triangle Pose involve bearing weight on the legs and hips, stimulating the bones and promoting bone growth. These poses engage the major muscle groups, including the legs, hips, and spine, providing an opportunity to strengthen the bones in these areas.

2. **Spinal Extension and Gentle Backbends**: Osteoporosis often affects the vertebrae of the spine, leading to a loss of height, curvature changes, and an increased risk of fractures. Yoga poses that focus on spinal extension and gentle backbends, such as Cobra Pose, Bridge Pose, and Sphinx Pose, help strengthen the back muscles, improve posture, and promote bone health in the spine.
3. **Core Strengthening:** A strong core is essential for maintaining stability and balance, reducing the risk of falls. Yoga poses that target the core, such as Boat Pose, Plank Pose, and Side Plank Pose, help strengthen the abdominal and back muscles, improving overall stability and supporting healthy posture.
4. **Balance and Coordination**: Osteoporosis increases the risk of falls, which can lead to fractures. Yoga poses that challenge balance, such as Tree Pose, Warrior III, and Eagle Pose, help improve proprioception and balance skills. Practicing these poses can enhance stability, body awareness, and coordination, reducing the likelihood of falls and injuries.

5. **Mindfulness and Stress Reduction:** Chronic stress and anxiety can contribute to bone loss and affect overall health. Yoga's emphasis on mindfulness, breathwork, and relaxation techniques can help reduce stress levels, promote a sense of calmness, and support overall well-being. By managing stress, you create a more conducive environment for optimal bone health.

Safe Modifications

If you have osteoporosis or osteopenia, it is essential to modify yoga poses to suit your specific needs. Avoid forward folds or twists that involve rounding the spine and putting pressure on the vertebrae. Opt for gentler variations that focus on lengthening and strengthening the muscles around the spine, rather than compressing it.

It is important to work with a knowledgeable yoga instructor who has experience in adapting poses for individuals with osteoporosis. They can guide you in selecting appropriate poses, modifications, and adaptations based on your bone health and personal limitations. It is also important to inform your instructor about your condition to ensure a safe and effective practice.

Remember to listen to your body and practice self-care. If a pose causes discomfort or pain, modify it or skip it altogether. Focus on gradual progress and work within your comfort zone. Regular and consistent practice, combined with proper nutrition and medical management, can contribute to improved bone health and overall well-being.

By incorporating yoga into your lifestyle, you can actively support your bone health, strengthen your body, improve balance, and reduce the risk of fractures. Embrace the transformative power of yoga as a tool to enhance your bone health and live a vibrant and active life.

Back Pain and Spine Health

Back pain is a common ailment that affects people of all ages, and it can significantly impact daily life, mobility, and overall well-being. Whether it's caused by poor posture, muscle imbalances, injury, or age-related changes, incorporating yoga into your routine can be an effective and holistic approach to managing back pain, improving spinal health, and promoting overall strength and flexibility.

Yoga offers a gentle and mindful way to address back pain and support spinal health. It focuses on strengthening the core muscles, improving posture, increasing flexibility, and promoting proper alignment. Through the practice of asanas (poses), pranayama (breathwork), and relaxation techniques, yoga can alleviate pain, reduce muscle tension, and enhance the stability and mobility of the spine.

Here are some key ways in which yoga can help with back pain and promote spinal health:

1. **Core Strengthening:** Weak core muscles can contribute to back pain and poor posture. Yoga poses such as Plank Pose, Boat Pose, and Bridge Pose target the abdominal and back muscles, strengthening the core and providing support for the spine. A strong core helps maintain proper alignment, reduces strain on the back, and improves overall stability.

2. **Spinal Alignment and Extension:** Yoga emphasizes proper spinal alignment and encourages the natural curves of the spine. Poses like Mountain Pose, Cat-Cow Stretch, and Cobra Pose promote spinal extension, improve posture, and alleviate muscle imbalances. These poses help counteract the effects of prolonged sitting, which often contributes to back pain.
3. **Flexibility and Range of Motion:** Tight muscles and limited range of motion can contribute to back pain. Yoga poses gently stretch and lengthen the muscles along the spine, hips, and legs, promoting flexibility and relieving tension. Poses such as Forward Fold, Triangle Pose, and Child's Pose target the hamstrings, lower back, and hips, providing relief and promoting suppleness in the spine.
4. **Gentle Twists and Backbends:** Controlled twists and gentle backbends in yoga can help release tension, improve spinal mobility, and alleviate back pain. Poses such as Seated Spinal Twist, Supported Bridge Pose, and Sphinx Pose gently rotate and extend the spine, promoting flexibility and creating space between the vertebrae.

5. **Relaxation and Stress Reduction:** Stress and emotional tension can contribute to muscle tightness and back pain. Yoga's focus on mindfulness, deep breathing, and relaxation techniques helps reduce stress levels, calm the nervous system, and relax the muscles. Practices such as Savasana (Corpse Pose), Yoga Nidra, and guided meditation can promote relaxation and relieve mental and physical tension.
6. **Proper Lifting and Body Mechanics:** Yoga teaches body awareness and proper alignment, which can be applied to daily activities, including lifting objects. By incorporating the principles of yoga into your movements, such as engaging the core, lifting with the legs, and maintaining a neutral spine, you can prevent unnecessary strain on the back and reduce the risk of injury.

It is important to approach yoga for back pain with patience, consistency, and awareness of your body's limitations. Start with gentle poses and gradually progress as your body becomes more comfortable and stronger. If you have specific back conditions or chronic pain, it is advisable to consult with a qualified yoga instructor or a healthcare professional who can guide you in choosing appropriate poses and modifications tailored to your needs.

Remember to listen to your body and practice self-care. If a pose exacerbates your back pain or feels uncomfortable, modify it or skip it altogether. Focus on finding a balance between challenge and comfort, and honor your body's limits. Regular practice, combined with proper posture, ergonomic adjustments, and healthy lifestyle habits, can contribute to long-term relief and support spinal health.

By incorporating yoga into your routine, you can find relief from back pain, improve spinal strength and flexibility, and cultivate a greater sense of well-being and vitality in your daily life. Embrace the transformative power of yoga as a tool to nurture your spine and restore harmony to your body and mind.

Modifying the Practice for Specific Conditions

Yoga is a versatile practice that can be modified to accommodate various health conditions and individual needs. Whether you're dealing with chronic pain, recovering from an injury, managing a specific medical condition, or simply have unique physical considerations, modifying the practice of yoga can help you reap its benefits while ensuring safety and comfort.

Modifications in yoga involve making adjustments to poses, using props, altering the intensity or duration of the practice, and incorporating variations that suit your specific condition or limitations. The goal is to create a practice that supports your well-being, addresses your specific needs, and respects the boundaries of your body.

Here are some common health conditions and considerations for which yoga can be modified:

Joint Conditions (Arthritis, Osteoarthritis, Rheumatoid Arthritis):

For individuals with joint conditions, it's important to avoid excessive stress on the joints and opt for gentle movements. Modify poses by reducing the range of motion, using props like blocks or blankets for support, and choosing poses that don't exacerbate joint pain. Focus on gentle stretches, range-of-motion exercises, and poses that promote joint mobility and circulation.

Back Pain and Spinal Issues (Herniated Disc, Scoliosis, Spinal Stenosis):

When dealing with back pain or spinal issues, it's crucial to prioritize proper alignment, spinal stability, and avoiding excessive strain on the affected areas. Modify poses by using props such as bolsters or straps to support the spine, avoid deep forward folds or twists that may aggravate the condition, and focus on gentle spinal stretches, core strengthening exercises, and poses that promote spinal elongation.

Cardiovascular Conditions (Hypertension, Heart Disease): If you have cardiovascular conditions, it's important to practice yoga in a controlled and mindful manner. Avoid intense or strenuous poses that may elevate blood pressure or put undue stress on the heart. Focus on gentle, restorative poses, mindful breathing techniques (such as diaphragmatic breathing), and relaxation practices that promote calmness and reduce stress levels.

Respiratory Conditions (Asthma, Chronic Obstructive Pulmonary Disease): Individuals with respiratory conditions should approach yoga with caution, especially when it comes to vigorous or strenuous practices that may trigger breathing difficulties. Modify poses to ensure proper breathing, avoid holding the breath, and incorporate gentle chest-opening poses, deep breathing exercises, and relaxation techniques that enhance lung capacity and promote relaxation.

Balance and Mobility Issues (Parkinson's Disease, Multiple Sclerosis): If you experience balance or mobility issues, focus on poses that improve stability, strengthen the lower body, and enhance coordination. Use props or a wall for support, practice seated or supported poses, and incorporate balance exercises that help improve proprioception and reduce the risk of falls. Adapt the practice to your abilities and embrace modifications that foster safety and confidence.

Remember, it's important to consult with a healthcare professional or a qualified yoga instructor when modifying your yoga practice for specific conditions. They can provide personalized guidance, suggest appropriate modifications, and help you create a practice that aligns with your needs and goals.

Listen to your body and practice self-care. Be aware of any discomfort or pain during the practice and modify or skip poses as needed. Honor your limits, progress gradually, and be patient with yourself. With the right modifications and a mindful approach, yoga can be a valuable tool in supporting your health, well-being, and personal journey towards balance and vitality.

Seeking Guidance from Healthcare Professionals

When it comes to incorporating yoga into your healthcare routine, seeking guidance from healthcare professionals is a crucial step to ensure a safe and effective practice. While yoga offers numerous benefits for physical and mental well-being, it is important to approach it in a way that complements and aligns with your overall healthcare plan. Consulting with medical professionals, such as your primary care physician, specialists, or physical therapists, can provide valuable insights and help you navigate the integration of yoga into your specific health context.

One of the primary reasons to seek guidance from healthcare professionals is to undergo a comprehensive assessment of your health status. These professionals have the knowledge and expertise to evaluate your medical history, current condition, and any potential contraindications or precautions that need to be considered when practicing yoga. By understanding your unique health profile, they can provide insights into the types of yoga practices that may be suitable for you and any modifications or adaptations that may be necessary to ensure a safe practice.

Healthcare professionals can offer individualized advice tailored to your specific needs. They can provide recommendations on the types of yoga practices that align with your condition, taking into account factors such as your fitness level, flexibility, and any existing physical limitations. This personalized guidance helps ensure that your yoga practice is optimized to support your health goals while minimizing the risk of injury or exacerbation of symptoms. They can suggest modifications or the use of props to accommodate your needs, enabling you to participate in yoga classes or practice at home with confidence.

Moreover, healthcare professionals can collaborate with yoga instructors or therapists to create a cohesive and holistic approach to your well-being. They can communicate relevant information about your health conditions, medications, or recent treatments to the yoga professionals, fostering an understanding of your specific requirements and ensuring that the yoga practice aligns with your overall healthcare plan. This collaborative effort promotes a team-based approach to your health and well-being, with healthcare professionals and yoga instructors working together to support your journey.

It is important to note that healthcare professionals may also provide guidance on when to avoid certain types of yoga or specific poses that could be contraindicated for your condition. For example, if you have a recent injury or are recovering from surgery, they may advise against certain movements or weight-bearing exercises until you have healed sufficiently. This guidance helps prevent potential complications and ensures that your yoga practice is conducted in a manner that is safe and appropriate for your individual circumstances.

By seeking guidance from healthcare professionals, you can feel empowered and confident in your yoga practice. They can offer reassurance, answer any questions or concerns you may have, and provide ongoing support as you progress in your yoga journey. Remember that healthcare professionals are there to support you in making informed decisions about your health, and their input is invaluable when it comes to integrating yoga into your overall healthcare plan.

Seeking guidance from healthcare professionals when incorporating yoga into your healthcare routine is essential. Their expertise, assessment, and individualized advice help ensure a safe and effective practice that aligns with your unique health needs. By collaborating with healthcare professionals, you can enhance the benefits of yoga while ensuring that your practice complements and supports your overall well-being.

Conclusion

Yoga can be a valuable tool for addressing common health issues and promoting overall well-being. Throughout this chapter, we explored various health conditions and how yoga can be adapted to support individuals dealing with joint stiffness and flexibility issues, arthritis and joint pain, osteoporosis and bone health concerns, as well as back pain and spinal health. We also discussed the importance of modifying the practice for specific conditions and seeking guidance from healthcare professionals.

By incorporating yoga into your healthcare routine, you can experience numerous benefits, including improved flexibility, strength, balance, reduced pain, enhanced relaxation, and a greater sense of overall well-being. The practice of yoga can be tailored to suit your individual needs, whether you're dealing with chronic pain, recovering from an injury, or managing specific medical conditions.

It is crucial to approach yoga for common health issues with mindfulness, patience, and self-awareness. Remember to listen to your body, honor your limitations, and practice self-care. Modify poses, use props, and adapt the practice to suit your specific needs and abilities. Seek guidance from healthcare professionals who can provide valuable insights and recommendations based on your unique health circumstances. Their expertise will help ensure a safe and effective integration of yoga into your healthcare routine.

As you embark on your yoga journey, remember that consistency and gradual progress are key. Embrace the transformative power of yoga as a holistic approach to managing and improving your health. With regular practice and the support of healthcare professionals, you can enhance your physical well-being, reduce discomfort, and cultivate a greater sense of balance, vitality, and inner peace.

Chapter 4: Yoga for Overall Well-being and Mindfulness

"Yoga is the art of creating space for yourself."
- Erich Schiffmann

Yoga is not just a physical practice; it is a holistic approach to nurturing your mind, body, and spirit. In this chapter, we will delve into the transformative power of yoga for overall well-being and mindfulness. Beyond the physical benefits, yoga offers a pathway to cultivate inner awareness, find balance, and connect with a deeper sense of self.

When we talk about overall well-being, we encompass not only the physical aspect but also mental and emotional wellness. Yoga provides a space for you to develop a greater sense of self-care and self-compassion, fostering a positive relationship with your body and mind. Through a combination of asanas (poses), pranayama (breathing techniques), and mindfulness practices, you can experience a profound sense of harmony and wholeness.

This chapter will explore various aspects of yoga that contribute to overall well-being and mindfulness. We will delve into the benefits of physical movement, explore the power of breath and its impact on the mind, and delve into mindfulness practices that bring awareness to the present moment. By integrating these elements into your yoga practice, you can enhance your overall well-being and cultivate a state of mindful living.

Throughout this chapter, we will explore the following topics:

Physical Movement: We will dive deeper into the physical aspect of yoga, exploring different asanas and their benefits for strength, flexibility, balance, and vitality. By incorporating these poses into your practice, you can improve your physical well-being, release tension, and increase energy flow throughout your body.

Pranayama (Breathing Techniques): Breath is an integral part of yoga practice. We will explore various pranayama techniques that help calm the mind, reduce stress, and enhance overall vitality. You will learn breathing exercises that can be incorporated into your daily life, allowing you to tap into a sense of inner peace and relaxation.

Mindfulness Practices: Mindfulness is the art of being fully present in the moment, cultivating awareness and acceptance without judgment. We will delve into mindfulness techniques such as meditation, body scanning, and mindful movement. These practices help you develop a greater sense of self-awareness, improve focus, and reduce stress, fostering a more balanced and centered approach to life.

By incorporating these elements into your yoga practice, you can experience a profound transformation in your overall well-being. You will develop a deeper connection between your mind, body, and breath, fostering a state of harmony and unity. As you embark on this journey of yoga for overall well-being and mindfulness, remember to approach the practice with an open mind, be patient with yourself, and embrace the process of self-discovery and growth.

So, let us embark on this exploration of yoga for overall well-being and mindfulness, and discover the immense benefits it holds for nurturing your mind, body, and spirit.

Stress Reduction and Relaxation

In our senior years, life may bring its own unique challenges and stressors. Physical changes, health concerns, and transitions in lifestyle can all contribute to increased stress levels. However, practicing yoga can be a valuable tool for seniors to reduce stress, cultivate relaxation, and enhance overall well-being. Yoga offers a gentle and accessible approach to stress reduction that can be adapted to suit the specific needs and abilities of seniors.

Let us explore how yoga can support seniors in managing stress and nurturing inner calm.

Gentle Asanas (Poses): Yoga for stress reduction in seniors focuses on gentle, supportive asanas that promote relaxation and release tension. These poses are specifically chosen to be safe and accessible for older bodies, considering any physical limitations or conditions. Gentle stretching, gentle twists, and seated poses can help improve circulation, release muscle tension, and induce a sense of physical relaxation. Through regular practice, seniors can experience increased flexibility, improved posture, and a greater sense of physical comfort, which all contribute to stress reduction.

Breathing Techniques (Pranayama): Pranayama, or breath control, is an essential aspect of yoga that can profoundly influence our state of mind and promote relaxation. Simple breathing exercises can be practiced by seniors to calm the mind, reduce stress, and bring a sense of balance and tranquility. Deep breathing techniques such as abdominal breathing, alternate nostril breathing, or extended exhale breathing can be particularly effective in inducing relaxation responses in the body. These techniques can be easily incorporated into daily routines or utilized during moments of stress to find immediate relief.

Mindfulness and Meditation: Mindfulness practices and meditation play a vital role in stress reduction and relaxation. Seniors can engage in mindfulness exercises that bring awareness to the present moment, fostering a sense of calm and inner peace. This can be as simple as focusing on the breath, observing sensations in the body, or practicing gratitude and loving-kindness. Regular meditation practice, even for short durations, can help seniors cultivate a deeper sense of relaxation, clarity, and overall well-being.

Restorative Yoga: Restorative yoga offers a nourishing and deeply relaxing practice for seniors. This style of yoga involves supported poses using props such as bolsters, blankets, and blocks, allowing the body to fully relax and let go of tension. Restorative poses are held for extended periods, creating an opportunity for seniors to experience profound physical and mental relaxation. These poses promote deep rest, rejuvenation, and restoration, offering a respite from the stresses of daily life.

Group Support and Community: Participating in yoga classes or joining a yoga community can provide seniors with a supportive and nurturing environment. Being part of a group with similar interests and goals can foster a sense of connection, belonging, and mutual support. Sharing the yoga journey with others can create a positive and uplifting atmosphere, enhancing the overall stress-reducing benefits of the practice.

As seniors engage in yoga for stress reduction and relaxation, it is important to listen to their bodies, honor their limitations, and practice self-care. It is recommended that seniors consult with healthcare professionals or experienced yoga instructors who can guide them in selecting appropriate poses and modifications based on their individual needs and conditions.

In conclusion, yoga offers seniors a powerful approach to reduce stress and cultivate relaxation. Through gentle asanas, breathing techniques, mindfulness practices, and restorative yoga, seniors can experience physical and mental relaxation, improved well-being, and a greater sense of inner calm. By integrating yoga into their daily lives, seniors can navigate the challenges of aging with grace, resilience, and a renewed sense of peace.

Mental Clarity and Focus

As we age, maintaining mental clarity and focus becomes increasingly important for our overall well-being. Yoga offers seniors a holistic approach to support cognitive health and enhance mental sharpness. By incorporating specific practices into their yoga routine, seniors can improve cognitive function, boost mental clarity, and cultivate a focused and alert mind. Let us explore how yoga can contribute to mental clarity and focus in the context of seniors.

Mind-Body Connection: Yoga emphasizes the integration of mind and body, fostering a deep connection between the two. Through the practice of asanas (poses) and mindful movement, seniors can enhance their body awareness and develop a stronger mind-body connection. This heightened awareness allows them to be fully present in the moment, cultivating focus and concentration.

Breathing Techniques: Pranayama, or breath control, is an integral part of yoga that has a direct impact on the mind. By practicing specific breathing techniques, seniors can regulate the breath, oxygenate the brain, and activate the relaxation response. Deep, controlled breathing can calm the mind, reduce stress, and enhance mental clarity and focus.

Meditation and Mindfulness: Regular meditation practice can significantly improve cognitive function, including attention span, memory, and mental clarity. Seniors can engage in various meditation techniques, such as focused attention or mindfulness meditation, to train the mind and enhance concentration. By bringing attention to the present moment and observing thoughts without judgment, seniors can develop mental resilience, improve focus, and promote mental clarity.

Balance and Coordination: Certain yoga poses and sequences require balance and coordination, which can challenge the mind and enhance cognitive function. By practicing balancing poses and movements that require coordination, seniors can sharpen their mental focus, improve proprioception (body awareness), and strengthen neural connections.

Brain-Boosting Poses: Certain yoga poses are known to stimulate the brain, increase blood flow, and enhance mental clarity. Poses like Downward Facing Dog, Headstand (with appropriate modifications), and Fish pose can invigorate the mind, improve circulation to the brain, and enhance mental alertness. Including these poses in the yoga routine can promote mental clarity and rejuvenation.

Social Interaction and Engagement: Participating in group yoga classes or joining a yoga community provides opportunities for social interaction and engagement. Interacting with others in a supportive and positive environment can stimulate the mind, foster mental engagement, and enhance cognitive function. Engaging in conversations, sharing experiences, and learning from others' perspectives can contribute to mental sharpness and focus.

Mindful Lifestyle Practices: In addition to the physical practice of yoga, incorporating mindful lifestyle practices into daily routines can support mental clarity. Seniors can integrate mindfulness into everyday activities such as eating, walking, and engaging in hobbies. Paying attention to the present moment, savoring experiences, and practicing mindfulness throughout the day can cultivate mental clarity and promote a focused mindset.

It is important for seniors to approach the practice of yoga for mental clarity and focus with patience and consistency. Each person's journey is unique, and progress may vary. Seniors should listen to their bodies, honor their limitations, and adapt the practice to suit their individual needs and abilities. Consulting with healthcare professionals or experienced yoga instructors can provide guidance and support in selecting appropriate practices and modifications.

In conclusion, yoga offers seniors a powerful means to enhance mental clarity, focus, and cognitive function. By integrating asanas, breathing techniques, meditation, and mindfulness practices into their yoga routine, seniors can sharpen their mental faculties, cultivate a focused mind, and promote overall cognitive well-being. Embracing yoga as a holistic practice can lead to a fulfilling and mentally vibrant senior journey.

Emotional Well-being and Self-Awareness

Emotional well-being is a vital aspect of overall health and happiness, and it becomes even more significant as we age. Yoga offers seniors a powerful path to cultivate emotional balance, enhance self-awareness, and nurture a deep sense of inner harmony. By integrating specific practices into their yoga routine, seniors can navigate the complexities of emotions, develop resilience, and foster a positive and empowered mindset.

Let us explore how yoga can support emotional well-being and self-awareness in the context of seniors.

Mindfulness and Self-Reflection: Yoga invites seniors to bring mindful awareness to their thoughts, feelings, and sensations. By practicing mindfulness, seniors can observe their emotions without judgment, allowing them to develop a deeper understanding of their inner world. This self-reflection enables seniors to recognize patterns, triggers, and reactions, empowering them to respond to emotions with greater clarity and compassion.

Emotional Release: Yoga provides a safe and supportive environment for emotional release. Through gentle movement, breathwork, and guided relaxation, seniors can release pent-up emotions, stress, and tension stored in the body. This cathartic process allows seniors to experience a sense of emotional relief, lightness, and renewal.

Breathwork for Emotional Regulation: The breath is a powerful tool for emotional regulation. Seniors can learn specific breathing techniques, such as deep belly breathing or calming breaths, to soothe the nervous system, reduce anxiety, and promote emotional balance. By consciously engaging with the breath, seniors can navigate and manage their emotions more effectively.

Heart-Opening Asanas: Certain yoga poses, such as backbends and chest-opening poses, can activate the heart center and facilitate emotional release and openness. These poses encourage seniors to connect with their emotions, cultivate self-compassion, and promote a sense of emotional well-being. Seniors can practice poses like Bridge pose, Camel pose, or Supported Fish pose to stimulate the heart center and access a deeper sense of emotional harmony.

Gratitude and Positive Affirmations: Incorporating gratitude practices and positive affirmations into their yoga routine can support seniors in fostering a positive mindset and cultivating emotional well-being. Seniors can engage in gratitude journaling, express appreciation for their body and life experiences, and repeat affirmations that uplift and inspire them. These practices can shift focus to the positive aspects of life, enhance self-esteem, and promote emotional resilience.

Restorative Yoga for Emotional Nourishment:
Restorative yoga offers seniors a deeply nourishing and calming practice. By practicing restorative poses supported by props, seniors can experience a profound relaxation response in the body, calming the mind and soothing emotions. These poses promote a sense of safety,

comfort, and emotional nourishment, allowing seniors to let go of stress and find emotional equilibrium.

Connection and Support: Engaging in yoga classes or joining a yoga community provides seniors with opportunities for connection, support, and emotional well-being. Being part of a community that shares similar values and goals can foster a sense of belonging and understanding. Seniors can share their yoga journey, connect with others, and receive support during times of emotional challenges.

It is essential for seniors to approach the practice of yoga for emotional well-being and self-awareness with gentleness and self-compassion. Each individual's emotional landscape is unique, and it is important to honor personal boundaries and triggers. Seniors should listen to their bodies, engage in practices that resonate with them, and seek guidance from healthcare professionals or experienced yoga instructors when needed.

In conclusion, yoga offers seniors a transformative path to cultivate emotional well-being, enhance self-awareness, and foster inner harmony. Through mindfulness, emotional release, breathwork, heart-opening poses, gratitude practices, restorative yoga, and connection, seniors can navigate their emotions with greater resilience and compassion. Embracing yoga as a holistic practice can support seniors in leading emotionally fulfilling and empowered lives.

Meditation and Mindfulness Techniques

Meditation and mindfulness are powerful practices that can profoundly impact seniors' well-being, promoting inner peace, mental clarity, and a deeper connection with the present moment. As part of the yoga journey, meditation and mindfulness techniques provide seniors with valuable tools to navigate the challenges of aging, enhance self-awareness, and cultivate a sense of calm and contentment. Let us explore how meditation and mindfulness can be integrated into the yoga practice for seniors.

Mindful Breathing: Mindful breathing is a foundational technique in meditation and mindfulness. Seniors can engage in focused breathing exercises, such as deep belly breathing or alternate nostril breathing, to anchor their attention to the breath. By directing attention to the sensations of breathing, seniors can cultivate present-moment awareness and develop a calm and centered state of mind.

Body Scan Meditation: Body scan meditation involves systematically directing attention to different parts of the body, noticing sensations, and cultivating a sense of embodied presence. Seniors can practice body scan meditation in a seated or lying-down position, slowly scanning through each body part with gentle awareness. This practice promotes relaxation, body awareness, and a deeper connection with the physical body.

Loving-Kindness Meditation: Loving-kindness meditation, also known as Metta meditation, is a practice that cultivates compassion and unconditional love towards oneself and others. Seniors can engage in loving-kindness meditation by silently repeating phrases of well-wishing, such as "May I be happy, may I be healthy, may I live with ease." This practice enhances self-compassion, kindness, and fosters a positive and inclusive mindset.

Guided Visualization: Guided visualization involves mentally picturing serene and calming scenes or engaging the imagination to create positive mental images. Seniors can follow guided meditations that lead them through visualizations of peaceful nature settings, healing imagery, or affirming experiences. This practice promotes relaxation, stress reduction, and enhances the mind's capacity for imagination and positive thinking.

Mindful Movement: Mindful movement, such as incorporating slow and deliberate movements in yoga sequences, can serve as a moving meditation. Seniors can practice mindful walking, Tai Chi, or gentle yoga flows with mindful attention to each movement, sensation, and breath. This practice cultivates a state of embodied awareness, grounding the mind in the present moment and fostering a sense of calm and mindfulness.

Mindfulness in Daily Activities: Yoga extends beyond the mat and into daily life. Seniors can integrate mindfulness into everyday activities by bringing awareness to routine actions such as eating, walking, or engaging in household chores. By engaging the senses, noticing sensations, and observing thoughts and emotions without judgment, seniors can infuse their daily activities with mindfulness and presence.

Silent Sitting Meditation: Silent sitting meditation involves sitting in stillness, observing the breath, thoughts, and sensations as they arise without attachment or judgment. Seniors can start with short periods of silent sitting meditation, gradually increasing the duration over time. This practice enhances focus, self-awareness, and the ability to cultivate inner stillness amidst the fluctuations of the mind.

It is important for seniors to approach meditation and mindfulness practices with patience, self-compassion, and a non-judgmental attitude. Each meditation session may be different, and it is important to embrace whatever arises without expectations. Seniors should find a comfortable meditation posture, create a peaceful environment, and integrate these practices into their daily routine at their own pace.

In summary, meditation and mindfulness techniques offer seniors profound opportunities to cultivate inner peace, presence, and self-awareness. By incorporating mindful breathing, body scan meditation, loving-kindness meditation, guided visualization, mindful movement, and silent sitting meditation into their yoga practice, seniors can experience a deepening of their spiritual journey and an enhanced quality of life.

Embracing Yoga Philosophy in Daily Life

Yoga is more than just a physical practice; it is a holistic way of life that offers profound insights and timeless wisdom to guide us on our journey of self-discovery and personal growth. For seniors, embracing yoga philosophy can be transformative, bringing greater meaning, harmony, and purpose to their daily lives. By integrating the principles and teachings of yoga philosophy into their thoughts, actions, and relationships, seniors can experience a deeper connection with themselves, others, and the world around them. Let us explore the essence of yoga philosophy and how seniors can embrace its wisdom in their everyday lives.

Living with Awareness and Mindfulness: Yoga philosophy teaches us the importance of living in the present moment and cultivating a state of awareness and mindfulness. Seniors can bring this practice into their daily lives by consciously savoring each experience, whether it be enjoying a cup of tea, engaging in a conversation, or appreciating the beauty of nature. By cultivating mindfulness, seniors can develop a deeper appreciation for the richness of life and find joy in the simplest of moments.

Practicing Gratitude and Contentment: Gratitude is at the core of yoga philosophy, reminding us to acknowledge and appreciate the abundance and blessings in our lives. Seniors can cultivate a gratitude practice by regularly reflecting on the things they are grateful for, whether it's their health, relationships, or the experiences that have shaped them. This practice fosters contentment, shifts the focus from what is lacking to what is present, and brings a sense of fulfillment and peace.

Embodying Non-Violence and Kindness: The principle of non-violence, known as ahimsa, encourages seniors to cultivate compassion, kindness, and empathy towards themselves and others. Seniors can practice ahimsa by treating themselves with gentleness and self-care, speaking words of kindness, and extending acts of compassion to those around them. Embracing non-violence fosters harmonious relationships, nurtures a positive environment, and creates a ripple effect of kindness in the world.

Cultivating Self-Acceptance and Self-Love: Yoga philosophy teaches us to embrace ourselves fully, accepting our strengths, weaknesses, and imperfections with love and compassion. Seniors can practice self-acceptance by letting go of self-judgment, appreciating their unique qualities, and nurturing a positive self-image. By cultivating self-love, seniors can experience a deep sense of worthiness, inner peace, and a genuine connection with their authentic selves.

Connecting with the Interconnectedness of All: Yoga philosophy emphasizes the interconnectedness of all beings and the interdependence of life. Seniors can embrace this principle by recognizing their connection to nature, animals, and other individuals. Engaging in acts of service, supporting environmental causes, or simply cultivating a sense of unity in their interactions can foster a profound sense of belonging and purpose.

Cultivating Equanimity and Letting Go: Yoga philosophy teaches us to cultivate equanimity, the ability to remain calm and balanced amidst the ups and downs of life. Seniors can practice equanimity by observing their reactions, accepting things they cannot change, and embracing the impermanence of life with grace. Cultivating equanimity allows seniors to navigate life's challenges with resilience, peace, and a sense of inner strength.

Nurturing a Connection with the Divine: Yoga philosophy acknowledges the presence of a higher power or divine consciousness within and around us. Seniors can nurture their spiritual connection through practices such as prayer, meditation, or contemplation. This connection provides solace, guidance, and a deeper sense of meaning, supporting seniors in finding purpose and transcending the limitations of the physical realm.

It is important for seniors to remember that embracing yoga philosophy is a personal journey, and each individual may resonate with different aspects of it. The key is to explore and integrate these teachings in a way that feels authentic and meaningful to them.

Embracing yoga philosophy in daily life offers seniors an opportunity to cultivate wisdom, harmony, and purpose. By living with awareness and mindfulness, practicing gratitude and contentment, embodying non-violence and kindness, cultivating self-acceptance and self-love, recognizing the interconnectedness of all, nurturing equanimity, and nurturing a connection with the divine, seniors can create a life of deep meaning, fulfillment, and inner peace. Yoga philosophy serves as a guiding light, empowering seniors to navigate the complexities of aging with grace, resilience, and a profound sense of purpose.

Self-Care Practices for Seniors

Self-care is a crucial aspect of maintaining overall well-being, especially for seniors. It involves taking intentional actions to nurture and prioritize one's physical, emotional, and mental health. Engaging in self-care practices allows seniors to enhance their quality of life, cultivate resilience, and promote a sense of self-worth and fulfillment. Let's explore a range of self-care practices specifically tailored for seniors, encompassing various aspects of their well-being.

Physical Self-Care

1. **Regular Exercise:** Engaging in regular physical activity tailored to individual abilities and interests promotes mobility, strength, and overall physical well-being. Seniors can participate in activities such as gentle yoga, walking, swimming, or tai chi to improve flexibility, cardiovascular health, and balance.
2. **Healthy Nutrition:** Nourishing the body with a well-balanced diet rich in fruits, vegetables, whole grains, and lean proteins supports optimal physical

health. Seniors should aim to consume nutrient-dense foods, stay hydrated, and limit the intake of processed foods and sugary beverages.
3. **Adequate Rest and Sleep**: Prioritizing sufficient rest and quality sleep is essential for seniors' overall health and vitality. Establishing a regular sleep routine, creating a comfortable sleep environment, and practicing relaxation techniques can promote restorative sleep

Emotional and Mental Self-Care

1. **Engaging in Hobbies and Interests:** Seniors should make time for activities they enjoy, whether it's reading, painting, gardening, or engaging in creative pursuits. These activities provide joy, fulfillment, and a sense of accomplishment.
2. **Social Connections:** Maintaining social connections and nurturing relationships is vital for emotional well-being. Seniors can engage in social activities, join clubs or groups of shared interests, or volunteer in their communities to foster meaningful connections and combat feelings of loneliness or isolation.

3. **Emotional Expression:** Seniors should prioritize emotional expression by acknowledging and processing their feelings. Engaging in activities such as journaling, practicing gratitude, or seeking therapy or counseling when needed can support emotional well-being.
4. **Stress Reduction Techniques:** Seniors can explore stress reduction techniques such as deep breathing exercises, meditation, mindfulness, or engaging in calming activities like nature walks or listening to soothing music. These practices promote relaxation, reduce anxiety, and improve overall mental well-being.

Spiritual Self-Care

1. **Meditation and Reflection:** Seniors can engage in meditation or reflective practices to nurture their spiritual well-being. This can involve moments of silence, connecting with nature, engaging in prayer, or participating in spiritual rituals that resonate with their beliefs and values.
2. **Engaging in Meaningful Practices**: Seniors can explore practices that bring them a sense of

purpose, such as volunteering, engaging in acts of kindness, or contributing to causes they care about. These activities foster a sense of connection, service, and spiritual fulfillment.
3. **Cultivating Inner Peace**: Seniors can prioritize moments of solitude, engage in activities that promote relaxation and introspection, and seek environments that inspire a sense of tranquility. These practices allow for inner reflection, centering the mind, and connecting with one's inner wisdom and peace.

Personal Care and Hygiene

Seniors should maintain good personal hygiene habits, including regular bathing, grooming, and oral care. It is essential to seek appropriate medical attention for any health concerns, maintain medication management, and attend regular check-ups with healthcare professionals.

Seeking Support and Assistance

It is crucial for seniors to recognize when they need support and seek assistance when necessary. This may involve reaching out to family, friends, or support networks for help, utilizing community resources for services like transportation or meal delivery, or seeking professional support from healthcare providers or therapists.

By embracing a holistic approach to self-care and implementing these practices into their daily lives, seniors can foster a sense of well-being, fulfillment, and empowerment. Engaging in physical self-care, nurturing emotional and mental well-being, cultivating spirituality, prioritizing personal care and hygiene, and seeking support when needed form the foundation for seniors to thrive and enjoy a vibrant and fulfilling life. Remember, self-care is an ongoing journey that requires self-awareness, self-compassion, and a commitment to nurturing oneself holistically.

Conclusion

Yoga serves as a powerful tool for promoting overall well-being and mindfulness in seniors. By integrating yoga into their lives, seniors can experience a multitude of physical, mental, and emotional benefits that contribute to their holistic health.

Through regular practice, seniors can enhance their physical fitness, improve flexibility, balance, and strength, and alleviate common health issues associated with aging. Yoga provides a gentle yet effective approach to exercise that can be tailored to individual needs, ensuring safety and comfort.

Beyond the physical benefits, yoga offers seniors a pathway to cultivate mindfulness and presence. The combination of movement, breath awareness, and meditation practices helps seniors develop a deep connection with their bodies and minds. This increased self-awareness fosters a greater understanding of one's thoughts, emotions, and overall well-being, leading to improved mental clarity, focus, and emotional balance.

Yoga also provides seniors with valuable tools for stress reduction and relaxation. By incorporating breathing techniques, meditation, and restorative poses into their practice, seniors can access a profound sense of calm and inner peace. These practices help to alleviate stress, anxiety, and depression, enhancing emotional well-being and promoting a positive outlook on life.

Furthermore, yoga philosophy encourages seniors to embrace values such as self-compassion, gratitude, and acceptance. This enables them to develop a kind and nurturing relationship with themselves and others, fostering emotional resilience, and promoting positive social connections.

It is important to note that yoga is a personal journey, and seniors should honor their bodies' limitations and practice at their own pace. Modifications and adaptations should be embraced to ensure a safe and enjoyable practice.

By integrating yoga into their daily lives, seniors can cultivate a greater sense of overall well-being, mindfulness, and self-empowerment. The benefits extend far beyond the physical realm, providing a holistic approach to health and vitality. Whether practiced on the mat or carried into everyday life, the principles of yoga offer seniors a pathway to live with intention, presence, and joy.

As seniors continue their yoga journey, they embark on a path of self-discovery, growth, and transformation. Through the regular practice of yoga, seniors have the opportunity to nurture their mind, body, and spirit, enhancing their overall well-being and embracing the gift of the present moment.

Chapter 5: Maintaining a Yoga Practice

"Yoga is the dance of every cell with the music of every breath that creates inner serenity and harmony."
- Debasish Mridha

Embarking on a yoga journey is a transformative experience, but the real essence lies in sustaining and maintaining a consistent practice over time. In this chapter, we will explore the key aspects of maintaining a yoga practice, including overcoming challenges, establishing a routine, and deepening your connection with yoga as a lifelong companion.

As we age, it becomes increasingly important to prioritize self-care and engage in activities that promote our physical, mental, and emotional well-being. Yoga offers a profound and accessible path to achieving and maintaining holistic health. However, maintaining a consistent practice requires commitment, perseverance, and an understanding of the factors that can either support or hinder our progress.

In this chapter, we will delve into strategies and insights that will help you overcome common obstacles and establish a sustainable yoga practice tailored to your needs as a senior. We will explore ways to navigate physical limitations, find motivation, adapt to changing circumstances, and deepen your connection with the practice. By addressing these aspects, you can ensure that yoga becomes an integral part of your life, providing lasting benefits and a sense of fulfillment.

Throughout the chapter, we will provide practical tips, guidance, and inspiration to support you on your journey of maintaining a yoga practice. Whether you are new to yoga or have been practicing for years, the insights shared here will help you stay motivated, navigate challenges, and continue reaping the benefits that yoga offers.

Remember, maintaining a yoga practice is not about perfection or achieving impressive physical feats. It is about showing up on your mat with an open heart and a willingness to connect with yourself, embracing the present moment as it unfolds. Your yoga practice is unique to you, and it will evolve as you grow and change. It is a constant exploration of self-discovery, self-care, and self-empowerment.

So, let's dive into the world of maintaining a yoga practice, where we will uncover the tools, strategies, and wisdom that will support you on your journey of sustaining a lifelong connection with yoga. By cultivating consistency, resilience, and a sense of curiosity, you can create a sustainable practice that nourishes your mind, body, and spirit, unlocking the transformative power of yoga in your everyday life

Establishing a Routine

Establishing a consistent routine is essential for maintaining a successful yoga practice. By creating a structured framework for your practice, you cultivate discipline, commitment, and a sense of regularity. Here are some valuable tips to help you establish a routine that supports your long-term engagement with yoga:

1. **<u>Set a Regular Practice Time:</u>** Determine a specific time of day that works best for you to practice yoga. It could be early morning, midday, or evening, depending on your schedule and personal preferences. Choose a time when you are least likely to be interrupted or distracted, allowing you to fully immerse yourself in your practice.

2. **<u>Create a Dedicated Space:</u>** Designate a dedicated space in your home where you can practice yoga. Clear the area of clutter, ensuring it is clean, inviting, and free from distractions. Decorate it with items that inspire and uplift you, such as candles, plants, or meaningful symbols. Having a designated space creates a sense of sacredness and helps to set the mood for your practice.

3. **<u>Start with Manageable Durations:</u>** When establishing your routine, begin with shorter practice sessions that are easily achievable. Starting with 10 to 15 minutes a day can be a great way to build consistency. As you become more

comfortable and your body adapts, gradually increase the duration of your practice. The key is to make it sustainable and enjoyable, rather than overwhelming yourself with long sessions that may lead to burnout.

4. **Plan Your Practice:** Outline a basic structure for your yoga practice. You may choose to focus on specific asanas (poses) or themes for each session. This provides a sense of direction and purpose, making your practice more intentional. Consider incorporating a warm-up, asanas, pranayama (breathing exercises), and relaxation or meditation into your routine.

5. **Find Accountability:** Accountability can play a significant role in maintaining a consistent yoga practice. Consider partnering with a friend or family member who shares your interest in yoga. You can practice together, share experiences, and hold each other accountable. Additionally, joining a yoga class or online community provides a supportive network of individuals who can motivate and inspire you on your yoga journey.

6. **Be Flexible:** While establishing a routine is important, it's also crucial to remain flexible and adaptable. Life can sometimes present unexpected challenges or disruptions. If you miss a scheduled practice, be gentle with yourself and return to your routine as soon as possible. Remember, yoga is a practice of compassion and self-care, and the intention behind your practice is what matters most.

By establishing a routine, you create a foundation for your yoga practice. It becomes an integral part of your daily life, allowing you to experience the multitude of benefits that yoga offers. Consistency cultivates a deeper connection with your body, mind, and spirit, enabling you to progress and grow on your yoga journey.

Adapting the Practice as You Age

As we age, our bodies naturally undergo changes, and it is essential to adapt our yoga practice to honor and support these changes. By modifying and adjusting our practice, we can continue to experience the benefits of yoga while respecting our evolving needs. Here are some valuable considerations for adapting your yoga practice as you age:

1. **Listen to Your Body:** As you engage in your yoga practice, pay close attention to how your body feels. Tune in to any sensations, discomfort, or limitations that may arise. It's crucial to listen to your body's wisdom and honor its messages. Modify or skip poses that cause pain or discomfort, and focus on those that feel safe and beneficial.

2. **Emphasize Gentle and Restorative Practices:** Gentle and restorative yoga styles can be particularly beneficial for seniors. These practices prioritize relaxation, flexibility, and nurturing the body. Gentle yoga styles, such as Hatha or Yin yoga, focus on slow and mindful movements, allowing you to explore your range of motion without strain. Restorative poses, supported by props, provide deep relaxation and rejuvenation, helping to release tension and calm the nervous system.

3. **Prioritize Balance and Stability:** Maintaining balance and stability becomes increasingly

important as we age. Incorporate poses that enhance balance, strengthen the core, and improve proprioception (awareness of body position). Tree pose, warrior poses, and standing balance poses are excellent for enhancing stability and cultivating a strong foundation.

4. **Adapt Poses to Your Needs:** Modify poses to suit your body's capabilities and limitations. Use props such as blocks, straps, and blankets to support and assist you in maintaining proper alignment and comfort. For instance, if you have limited mobility or flexibility, using a chair for seated poses or using a wall for support in standing poses can be immensely helpful. Adaptations allow you to experience the intended benefits of each pose while ensuring safety and comfort.

5. **Cultivate Mindful Movement:** As you age, it becomes even more crucial to practice yoga mindfully, focusing on the breath, alignment, and sensations in your body. Slow down and move with awareness, paying attention to your body's signals. Mindful movement not only reduces the risk of injury but also deepens your connection with the

present moment and enhances the meditative aspects of your practice.

6. **<u>Practice Self-Compassion:</u>** Embrace self-compassion and let go of any expectations or comparisons. Each individual's yoga journey is unique, and it's important to honor and accept your own progress and limitations. Remember that yoga is not about achieving perfect poses but about cultivating a sense of well-being and inner peace.

By adapting your yoga practice to accommodate your changing needs, you can continue to enjoy the numerous physical, mental, and emotional benefits of yoga as you age. Stay attuned to your body, be gentle with yourself, and approach your practice with an open heart and a sense of curiosity. Yoga is a lifelong journey of self-discovery, and adapting your practice allows you to embrace the transformative power of yoga at every stage of life.

Continuing Education and Growth

Yoga is a vast and ever-evolving practice, and as you maintain your yoga journey, it's important to prioritize continuing education and personal growth. By expanding your knowledge and exploring new aspects of yoga, you can deepen your understanding, refine your skills, and keep your practice fresh and inspiring. Here are some valuable considerations for continuing education and growth in your yoga practice:

1. **Attend Workshops and Retreats:** Participating in workshops and retreats led by experienced teachers offers a valuable opportunity to learn from different perspectives and deepen your practice. These immersive experiences provide focused teachings on specific aspects of yoga, such as meditation, pranayama, philosophy, or advanced asanas. Engaging in workshops and retreats can reinvigorate your practice and expand your understanding of yoga.

2. **Explore Advanced Training Programs:** If you wish to deepen your knowledge and become a

certified yoga teacher, consider enrolling in advanced training programs. These programs offer in-depth studies on yoga philosophy, anatomy, sequencing, and teaching methodologies. Advanced training programs not only enhance your personal practice but also equip you with the skills to guide and inspire others on their yoga journeys.

3. **Engage in Self-Study:** Dedicate time to self-study by exploring yoga literature, philosophical texts, and online resources. Reading books written by renowned yoga masters and scholars can provide valuable insights into the philosophy and principles of yoga. Additionally, there are numerous online platforms, podcasts, and blogs that offer educational content and discussions on various yoga-related topics.

4. **Connect with Experienced Teachers:** Seek guidance and mentorship from experienced yoga teachers. They can offer personalized advice, share their wisdom, and help you refine your practice. Attend classes taught by different teachers to gain diverse perspectives and learn from their unique teaching styles.

5. **Embrace a Beginner's Mindset:** Approach your practice with a beginner's mindset, maintaining a sense of curiosity and openness. Cultivate a willingness to explore new poses, techniques, and styles. Even if you have been practicing for years, there is always more to discover and learn. Embracing a beginner's mindset allows you to approach each practice with freshness and receptivity.

6. **Reflect and Journal:** Take time to reflect on your yoga journey and journal about your experiences. Reflecting on the effects of your practice, insights gained, and challenges faced helps deepen your self-awareness and understanding of the transformative power of yoga. Journaling can serve as a valuable tool for self-reflection, tracking your progress, and setting intentions for your ongoing growth.

By prioritizing continuing education and personal growth in your yoga practice, you ensure that your journey remains vibrant and meaningful. Remember, yoga is a lifelong exploration that goes beyond physical poses. It is a profound path of self-discovery, self-care, and self-transformation. Embrace the opportunities for learning, be open to new experiences, and allow your practice to evolve with grace and authenticity.

Finding Supportive Communities

Practicing yoga can be a transformative and enriching experience, especially when you surround yourself with supportive communities that share your passion for yoga. Connecting with like-minded individuals and being part of a supportive yoga community can enhance your practice, provide motivation, and foster a sense of belonging. Here are some valuable considerations for finding supportive communities in your yoga journey:

1. **Join Local Yoga Studios:** Explore and join local yoga studios in your area. Yoga studios often offer a variety of classes, workshops, and events that cater to different levels and interests. By becoming a member of a yoga studio, you gain access to a community of practitioners and teachers who share your dedication to the practice. Engaging in classes

together and connecting with fellow yogis can create a sense of camaraderie and mutual support.

2. **<u>Attend Community Events and Meetups:</u>** Keep an eye out for community events and yoga meetups in your area. These events may include outdoor yoga sessions, yoga festivals, or group meditation gatherings. Participating in these events allows you to connect with a diverse range of individuals who share a common interest in yoga. It's an opportunity to expand your network, exchange insights, and build connections with fellow yoga enthusiasts.

3. **<u>Online Yoga Communities:</u>** In today's digital age, online yoga communities and social media platforms provide avenues for connecting with a global network of yogis. Join online forums, Facebook groups, or follow yoga-related hashtags on platforms like Instagram. Engaging in these online communities enables you to interact with practitioners and teachers from around the world, share experiences, seek advice, and find inspiration.

4. **<u>Seek Out Yoga Retreats and Workshops</u>**: Yoga retreats and workshops are not only opportunities for personal growth but also

incredible platforms for connecting with like-minded individuals. These immersive experiences bring together individuals who are passionate about yoga, wellness, and self-discovery. The shared experience of practicing yoga, engaging in workshops, and enjoying mindful activities creates a nurturing and supportive environment for building lasting connections.

5. **Volunteer or Teach:** Consider volunteering at yoga events or community outreach programs. Offering your time and skills allows you to contribute to the yoga community while forming meaningful connections with fellow volunteers and participants. If you feel inspired, you may even explore the possibility of sharing your own knowledge and experiences by teaching yoga classes, particularly for seniors or specific groups with unique needs.

6. **Create Your Own Yoga Circle:** If you are unable to find a supportive community in your immediate surroundings, consider forming your own yoga circle. Gather a group of friends, neighbors, or fellow seniors who are interested in practicing yoga.

Arrange regular meetups where you can practice together, share insights, and support each other's growth. Creating your own community brings the opportunity to tailor the practice to your specific needs and create a supportive environment that aligns with your shared values.

Finding supportive communities in your yoga journey not only enhances your practice but also enriches your overall well-being. These communities provide spaces for growth, learning, and connection with individuals who understand and appreciate the transformative power of yoga. Remember, yoga is not only an individual practice but also a collective experience. By engaging with supportive communities, you nurture your own growth while contributing to the growth of others on the yoga path.

Conclusion

Maintaining a yoga practice is a lifelong commitment that offers numerous physical, mental, and emotional benefits. As you navigate your yoga journey, it is essential to establish a routine, adapt the practice as you age, prioritize continuing education and growth, find supportive communities, and implement tips for long-term success. By incorporating these elements into your practice, you can create a sustainable and fulfilling yoga journey.

Establishing a routine provides structure and consistency, allowing you to make yoga an integral part of your daily life. Adapting the practice as you age ensures that it remains accessible and beneficial, taking into consideration your body's changing needs and limitations. Continual learning and growth keep your practice fresh, inspiring, and aligned with the deeper aspects of yoga philosophy.

Finding supportive communities nurtures a sense of belonging, provides motivation, and offers opportunities for connection and growth with fellow practitioners. These communities create an environment of shared learning, support, and inspiration. Additionally, seeking guidance from experienced teachers and mentors contributes to your personal development and enriches your practice.

To maintain a yoga practice in the long term, it is crucial to implement tips for long-term success. This includes setting realistic goals, listening to your body, practicing self-care, and celebrating progress rather than focusing solely on outcomes. It also involves embracing patience and resilience, understanding that yoga is a journey of self-discovery and transformation that unfolds over time.

Remember, maintaining a yoga practice is not just about physical postures; it is a holistic path that encompasses breathwork, mindfulness, philosophy, and self-reflection. By prioritizing your practice, you cultivate a deeper connection with yourself, foster overall well-being, and embrace the transformative power of yoga.

As you embark on this journey, allow yourself the flexibility to adapt your practice, explore new avenues, and embrace the continuous evolution that comes with aging and personal growth. Embrace the challenges, celebrate the milestones, and remain open to the profound possibilities that yoga offers.

May your yoga practice continue to bring you strength, joy, and inner peace as you navigate the ever-unfolding path of self-discovery and well-being.

Conclusion

Throughout this book, we have delved into the world of yoga for seniors above 60, exploring its immense potential for enhancing physical well-being, promoting mental clarity, and fostering a deep sense of inner peace. As we conclude this journey, let's take a moment to recap the key points we have covered and reflect on the valuable insights gained.

We began by understanding the benefits of yoga for seniors. We explored how yoga can improve flexibility, strength, balance, and overall mobility, helping to alleviate common age-related issues. We also recognized its positive impact on mental health, stress reduction, and promoting a sense of overall well-being.

Addressing concerns and misconceptions, we highlighted the importance of dispelling any doubts or fears surrounding yoga practice for seniors. By acknowledging and addressing potential limitations and modifications, we create a safe and inclusive space where seniors can experience the transformative power of yoga.

Next, we delved into the practical aspects of practicing yoga for seniors. We explored essential equipment and props that can enhance comfort and support during the practice. We also discussed the significance of creating a dedicated yoga space, a personal sanctuary where seniors can immerse themselves in their practice and experience tranquility.

Moving forward, we explored different categories of yoga poses specifically tailored for seniors. We explored gentle warm-up exercises to prepare the body, standing poses to enhance stability and strength, seated poses to improve flexibility and posture, supine and prone poses to promote relaxation and release tension, balance poses to improve stability and coordination, and restorative poses to foster deep relaxation and rejuvenation.

Understanding that yoga can be adapted to address common health issues, we delved into specific conditions such as joint stiffness and flexibility, arthritis and joint pain, osteoporosis and bone health, as well as back pain and spinal health. We explored modifications and tailored approaches to ensure safety and maximum benefit for seniors with these conditions.

Embracing the holistic nature of yoga, we delved into the importance of mindfulness, breathing techniques, and meditation. We recognized how these practices can enhance mental clarity, reduce stress, and cultivate self-awareness. We also explored the philosophy behind yoga and how it can be integrated into daily life, leading to a more balanced and purposeful existence.

Moreover, we highlighted the significance of maintaining a yoga practice over time. We discussed the establishment of a routine, adaptation to the changing needs of the body as we age, the importance of continuous education and growth, finding supportive communities, and implementing tips for long-term success. These elements ensure that yoga remains a lifelong journey of self-discovery, growth, and well-being.

As we conclude this book, let us remember that yoga is a personal and transformative practice that can enrich every stage of life, including the senior years. It offers not only physical benefits but also mental and spiritual nourishment. By embracing yoga for seniors, we honor our bodies, cultivate self-awareness, and connect with the essence of who we are.

May the wisdom shared in this book serve as a guiding light on your yoga journey, empowering you to embrace the practice, explore its vast potential, and experience the profound benefits it offers. May your yoga practice continue to be a source of joy, well-being, and connection as you navigate the beautiful path of yoga for seniors above 60.

Printed in Great Britain
by Amazon